W9-BHV-419

The Practicing Physician's Approach to Headache

3rd EDITION

The Practicing Physician's Approach to Headache

3rd EDITION

Seymour Diamond, M.D.

Director, Diamond Headache Clinic
Chicago, Illinois
Adjunct Clinical Associate Professor of Neurology
The Chicago Medical School
Executive Officer, Research Group on Migraine
and Headache, World Federation of Neurology

Donald J. Dalessio, M.D.

Chairman, Department of Medicine
Scripps Clinic and Research Foundation
La Jolla, California
Clinical Professor of Neurology
University of California, San Diego

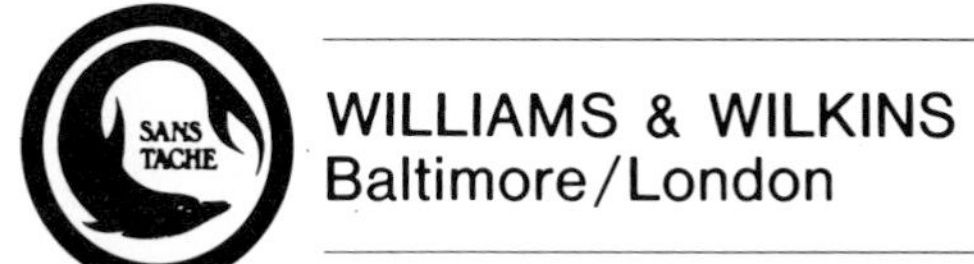

WILLIAMS & WILKINS
Baltimore/London

Made in the United States of America

Second Edition, 1978
Reprinted 1979

Library of Congress Cataloging in Publication Data

Diamond, Seymour, 1925–
The practicing physician's approach to headache.

Bibliography: p.
Includes index.
1. Headache. I. Dalessio, Donald J., 1931– . II. Title. [DNLM: 1. Headache. WL 342 D537p]
RC392.D53 1982 616.8′49 81-19645
ISBN 0-683-02503-1 AACR2

Composed and printed at the
Waverly Press, Inc.
Mt. Royal and Guilford Aves.
Baltimore, Md 21202, U.S.A.

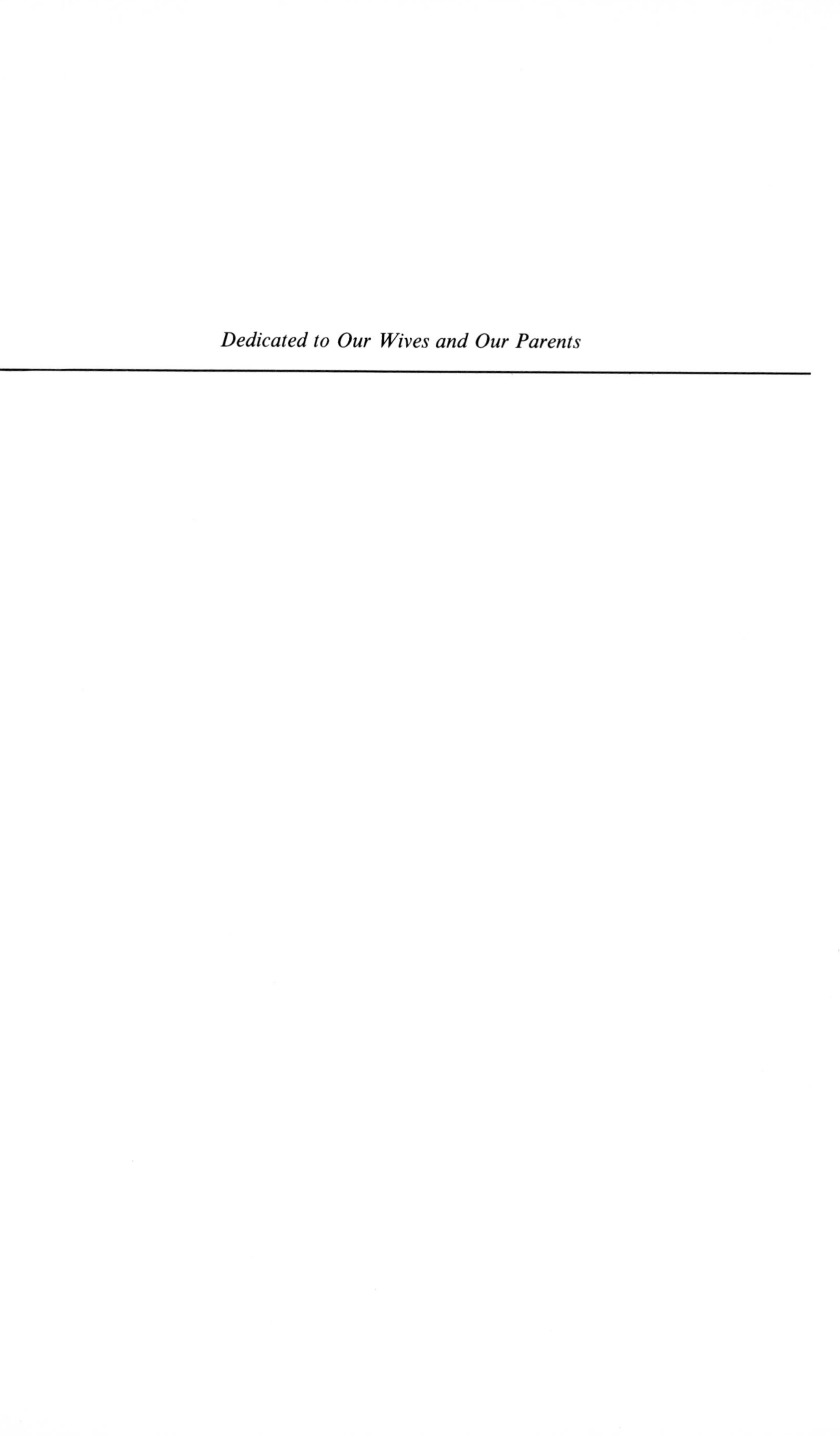

Dedicated to Our Wives and Our Parents

Preface to the Third Edition

"Horses for courses," say the racetrack touts.

And so it is with books. This book, now in its third edition, is created for one consumer, the practitioner of medicine. Since headache is so commonplace, almost all active practitioners are liable to be faced with large numbers of patients with headache as their chief complaint, especially those engaged in primary or community medicine, in the outpatient practice of medicine. Hopefully, this book will fill their needs.

Our continuing goals have been to tailor the manuscript to stress simplicity and directness. When necessary, repetition is employed for emphasis. We like to term this book a "working text," actively employed by its purchasers and adaptable to various clinical situations. Deliberately, we have not attempted to be comprehensive or exhaustive or to cover occult causes of head pain.

Several minor changes have been made; we have omitted the brief tests at the end of each chapter, have placed references of a useful nature at the end of each chapter, and have placed an Atlas of drawings by Frank Netter, M.D. at the end of the written text for added emphasis.

Preface to the First Edition

Two important factors are paramount in the treatment and management of headache patients. The first is that perhaps half of them have been treated symptomatically—without regard to a diagnosis and with drugs used simply to relieve pain. There should be a logical sequence employed in investigating the problem. Many headache patients have not had a careful history or neurologic examination, nor has an adequate attempt been made to diagnose the type of cephalalgia from which they suffer. Even though the history and neurologic examination are the keys to the diagnosis, extensive testing procedures may have been performed without discrimination. It is the intention of the authors to promote and provide a logical understanding of the headache patient and the approach to the diagnosis and treatment of his problem.

To the patient who has suffered over a long period of time, his headache is most important, not "just a headache." He will travel from doctor to doctor and to large research and diagnostic centers. This brings us to our second important point. Diagnosis must be coordinated with continual treatment. The cephalalgic patient needs attention and treatment on a continuing basis, whether the diagnosis indicates psychogenic, vascular or organic causes. The follow-up treatment may be on the basis of trial and error until relief is afforded. Therefore, the patient must have full confidence in his physician and his approach to the problem. It is easier for one physician to mold his confidence rather than a continued series of consultants.

We should not, as physicians, be intolerant of the headache sufferer. It is easy to lose patience and lack concern for these people, especially those with persistent complaints. The simplest course is to blame the problem on a defective personality or the wish of the patient to avoid reality. Careful attention to symptoms and related details, however, will reveal the etiology and guide the subsequent treatment.

It is not the purpose of this book to be a reference text giving a multitude of information. Rather, we hope to demonstrate a definitive approach to both the diagnosis and the treatment of headache. An attempt has been made to keep the text uncluttered, simple and easy to read and follow.

About the Authors

Seymour Diamond, MD, Adjunct Clinical Associate Professor of Neurology, the Chicago Medical School, and Director, Diamond Headache Clinic, Ltd., Chicago, Illinois, received his MD degree from the Chicago Medical School. His internship and residencies were spent in Little Rock University Hospital in Arkansas and White Cross Hospital, Columbus, Ohio. He is past president of the American Association for the Study of Headache and of the National Migraine Foundation. Dr. Diamond has published numerous articles on headache and is a frequent lecturer on this subject. He is currently executive officer of the Research Group on Migraine and Headache, World Federation of Neurology.

Donald J. Dalessio, MD, matriculated at Wesleyan and Yale and trained in Neurology and Medicine at New York Hospital-Cornell Medical Center and at Yale. Dr. Dalessio is presently Chairman, Department of Medicine, Scripps Clinic and Research Foundation, La Jolla, California, and Clinical Professor of Neurology, University of California, San Diego School of Medicine. He is editor of the journal *Headache* and author of *Wolff's Headache and Other Head Pain*, 3rd and 4th editions.

Acknowledgments

We are particularly indebted to Judi Falk for illustrations for this work; to Joseph R. Kraft, MD, Chairman, Department of Clinical Pathology and Nuclear Medicine, St. Joseph Hospital, Chicago, Illinois, for his help with the scanning section of the book; Robert J. Borgerson, MD, Chairman, Radiology Department, St. Joseph Hospital, Chicago, Illinois, for the x-ray illustrations; Harvey Lee Meyers, Jr., MD, Associate Professor of Neurology, the Chicago Medical School, Chicago, Illinois, for his help with certain illustrative material; Bernard J. Baltes, MD, PhD, our co-worker in headache and Martin E. Bruetman, MD, Professor and Chairman, Department of Neurology, the Chicago Medical School, Chicago, Illinois.

We acknowledge our debt to others who work in this field, and whose names appear in the bibliography. In particular, the painstaking and careful work of the late Harold G. Wolff, MD, deserves mention.

Special mention should also be given to Mrs. Betty Stewart of Chicago and Mrs. Joan Bryan of Lexington for their help in the preparation of this manuscript.

For the 2nd edition, Catherine Dalessio has revised some of the drawings. We thank Mrs. Camille Mead, of La Jolla, for help with the manuscript preparation. Drs. Stanley Seat and James Usselman of Scripps Clinic have prepared new radiographs including computerized tomographic scans. Mrs. Ruby Richardson of Williams & Wilkins coordinated the project as Editor.

For the 3rd edition, we have used illustrations which were completed by Dr. Frank Netter for the *CIBA Symposium* issue on "Headaches." Ms. Barbara Bekiesz and Ms. Ellin Mair of the *CIBA Symposium* have also assisted in this matter. R. Robert Erickson, M.D., University of Chicago Hospitals, Chicago, Illinois has assisted in the preparation of this manuscript. We would also like to thank Ms. Norma McEwen for her editorial assistance.

If a writer is so cautious that he never writes anything that cannot be criticized, he will never write anything that can be read. If you want to help other people you have got to make up your mind to write things that some men will condemn.

Thomas Merton
"Seeds of Contemplation"

Contents

1

Classification and Mechanisms of Headache

Since all physicians may be called upon to treat patients with headache, it is important to have a simple classification which may give clues to appropriate therapy. We have separated headache into three main groups, rather than providing a series of disparate headache syndromes which may tax the memory. These groups are *vascular*, *muscle contraction* and *traction and inflammatory* (Table 1.1).

Vascular headache includes classic and common migraine, hemiplegic and ophthalmoplegic migraine, cluster headache, toxic vascular headache and hypertensive headache. Common to all these is a tendency to vascular dilation, which provokes the headache phase in each instance. Vasoconstriction may also occur and may be responsible for the painless sensory and motor phenomena occurring with some forms of vascular headache. Toxic vascular headache refers to that state evoked by a systemic vasodilation and may be produced by fever, ingestion of alcohol, poisons, CO_2 retention, and therapeutic agents such as the nitrates. Hypertensive headache is related to elevation in the systemic arterial blood pressure.

Perhaps the most common form of headache is that termed "muscle contraction headache" and is characterized by persistent contraction of the muscles of the head, neck and face. This produces dull, bandlike, persistent pain, which may last for days, months or years. When the headache is incapacitating, persistent and not obviously vascular in nature, a disorder of mood, thought or behavior should be suspected. This complaint is frequently seen in the depressed patient but is not exclusively associated with depression. Headache may also be a sign of chronic anxiety or may present as a form of a contemporary conversion reaction.

Traction and inflammatory headache includes headache evoked by organic diseases of the skull or its components, including the brain, meninges, arteries, veins, eyes, ears, teeth, nose and paranasal sinuses. The term "traction headache" is used to describe the often nonspecific headache seen with mass lesions of the brain, including tumors, hematomas, abscesses, and brain edema for whatever cause. Traction and inflammatory headache of a particularly intense type occurs in subarachnoid hemorrhage. Traction and inflammatory headache is associated with inflammatory disease of the meninges and with intracranial or extracranial arteritis or phlebitis. Inflammatory headache may be associated with disease of the special sense organs and the teeth and with disorders of the joints of the neck and the jaw. The major neuralgias are also listed here, in parentheses, since the neuritic pain which characterizes these conditions is associated with specific abnormalities of the function of the central nervous system.

The management of traction and inflammatory headache or the major neuralgias generally involves specific treatment for the associated underlying disease. The patient whose headache is classified in this group may require extensive investigation and numerous consultations with neurologists, neurosurgeons, ophthalmologists, otolaryngologists and dentists. Thus, treatment for this form of headache or facial pain is extremely varied and may range from surgery to anticonvulsants. It is in this group that prompt and emergency treatment is often required; the headache or facial pain is considered a secondary phenomenon, which often responds to alleviation of the primary disease.

All the conditions mentioned above and listed in the classification of headache will be discussed in detail in subsequent chapters.

Table 1.1. Classification and Treatment of Headache*

Vascular Headache	Muscle Contraction Headache	Traction and Inflammatory Headache
Migraine Classic Common Hemiplegic } complicated Ophthalmoplegic } migraine Cluster (histamine) Toxic vascular Hypertensive	Depressive equivalents and conversion reactions Cervical osteoarthritis Chronic myositis	Mass lesions (tumors, edema, hematomas, cerebral hemorrhage) Diseases of the eye, ear, nose, throat, teeth Arteritis, phlebitis (cranial neuralgias) Occlusive vascular disease Atypical facial pain TMJ disease
	Suggested Treatment	
Ergot derivatives Sedation Methysergide Cyproheptadine Propranolol Clonidine Lithium Platelet antagonist Analgesics Antihypertensives Behavioral conditions	Common analgesics Sedation Antidepressants Physical therapy Behavioral conditioning	Appropriate consultation Therapy of underlying disease Antibiotics } Anticonvulsants } Corticosteroids } as indicated Miotics } Surgery }

* Ad Hoc Committee, 1962.

wrong pace or wrong direction rather than a structural disease of the nervous system. Nonetheless, headache may also be the presenting complaint in catastrophic illness such as brain tumor, cerebral hemorrhage or meningitis, and to ignore the symptom in this context is to risk the life of the patient. Headache may be intense whether its source is benign or malignant. The problem is compounded further by the difficulties involved in studying the brain and its appendages, which are encased in the bony fortress of the skull and resist the usual efforts of diagnosis. It forces one to rely on peripheral methods of investigation.

THE NATURE OF HEADACHE

Knowledge of headache and its variants is essential to the practitioner. Headache is a unique syndrome in medicine and has been termed the most common medical complaint of civilized man. Yet severe headache is only infrequently caused by organic disease. Hence, it may be inferred that for the most part headache represents an inability of the individual to deal in some measure with the uncertainties of life—that it is a symptom of

ANATOMIC SUBSTRATE OF PAIN

What structures of the head are capable of causing pain? In a series of anatomic studies, performed for the most part on patients prepared for neurologic surgery, Ray and Wolff (1940) showed that the pain-sensitive structures of the head include the skin of the scalp and its blood supply and appendages, the head and neck muscles, the great venous sinuses and their tributaries, parts of the dura mater at the base of the brain, the dural arteries, the intracerebral arteries, at least the fifth, sixth and seventh cranial nerves and the cervical nerves. The cranium, the brain parenchyma, much of the dura and pia mater, the ependymal lining of the ventricles and the choroid plexuses are not sensitive to pain (Table 1.2).

appropriate, since vasodilation in itself does not invariably produce headache. One does not usually complain of headache, for example, after severe exertion or after sitting in a tub of hot water. Yet extracranial vasodilation is obvious at these times. Thus it has been suggested that the peripheral manifestations of migraine (or, as the patient describes it, the "pounding headache") are related to vasodilation associated with a sterile local inflammatory reaction. In other terms, it has been suggested that migraine is a clinical syndrome of self-limited neurogenic inflammation.

Table 1.2. Pain Sensitivity of Cranial Tissues

	Pain Sensitive	Insensitive to Pain
Intracranial	Cranial sinuses and afferent veins Arteries of the dura mater Arteries of the base of the brain and their major branches Parts of the dura mater (in the vicinity of large vessels)	Parenchyma of the brain Ependyma, choroid plexus Pia mater, arachnoid membrane, parts of the dura mater
Extracranial	Skin, scalp, fascia, muscles Mucosa Arteries (veins: less sensitive)	Skull (periosteum slightly sensitive)
Nerves	Trigeminal, facial, vagal, glossopharyngeal 2nd and 3rd cervical nerves	

In general, pain pathways for structures above the tentorium cerebelli are contained in the trigeminal nerve, and pain that is referred from these structures is usually appreciated in the frontal, temporal and parietal regions of the skull. Pain pathways for structures below the tentorium cerebelli are contained especially in the glossopharyngeal and vagus nerves, as well as the upper cervical spinal roots. Pain referred from these structures is usually felt in the occipital region of the head.

THE BIOCHEMISTRY OF MIGRAINE

In order to understand the roles of the vasoactive substances in migraine, a brief discussion of some mechanisms of inflammation is necessary. See Plate 14.2, Chapter 14. This is

Vasodilation alone does not invariably produce headache. Probably, inflammation is involved also.

Furthermore, when one begins to study inflammation one must also study blood clotting, the complement system and immune mechanisms, for all the systems are intertwined. Indeed, their separation is unnatural.

Inflammation begins with a series of cellular events (Movat, 1972). Usually a specific or nonspecific injury occurs, provoked by multiple factors including ischemia or injury, the deposition of immune complexes, activation of the Hageman factor, deposition of bacterial toxins and, possibly, stress and/or higher nervous activity. Vasoactive amines such as histamine and serotonin are released from platelets, basophils and tissue mast cells. Other tissues, when injured, may release slow-reacting substance of anaphylaxis (SRSA) and prostaglandins. All are vasoactive and increase vascular permeability. Serum components come in contact with extravascular proteins, modifying these proteins. The complement cascade is stimulated (Müller-Eberhard, 1977). Fixation of complement, for example to immune complexes, attracts polymorphonuclear leukocytes which localize in the area. Upon rupture of the lysosomal membranes of the leukocytes, a series of enzymes are elaborated. Kinins are produced when the coagulation system is activated. Prostaglandins are released by antigen-antibody reactions and by bradykinin; prostaglandins themselves aggregate platelets, causing their disruption and so increasing the concentration of vasoactive substances.

Thus, present evidence implicates at least five and possibly more groups of vasoactive substances associated with inflammation, including

- catecholamines
- histamine and serotonin
- peptide kinins
- prostaglandins
- slow-reacting substance of anaphylaxis (SRSA), an acidic lipid.

All have potent biologic properties which differ with their structure and include among other effects

- contraction and relaxation of smooth muscle
- constriction or dilation of arteries and veins
- induction of water and sodium diuresis
- fever
- wheal-and-flare reactions
- induction of pain, including headache

The migraine episode can be studied only in humans, and its study is limited by its relatively benign course and the lack of a suitable animal experimental model. Nonetheless, the following statements about vasoactive substances as they affect the migraine episode may be made:

- Serotonin levels fall at onset of migraine.
- Local accumulation of a vasodilator polypeptide occurs.
- Tyramine taken orally may evoke migraine.
- Temporal arteries of migrainous patients bind norepinephrine.
- Injected prostaglandins evoke vascular headache.
- Histamine levels are increased in cluster headache.

Serotonin levels of the plasma fall at the onset of a migraine attack and platelets of patients with migraine, incubated with serotonin, aggregate more readily than those of controls. Serotonin will constrict scalp arteries in man. An increase in the major metabolite of serotonin, 5-hydroxyindole-acetic acid (5HIAA), has been inconsistently demonstrated during a migraine attack (Anthony et al., 1969; Sicuteri, 1967).

Deshmukh and Meyer (1977) investigated the pathophysiologic role of platelets in the pathogenesis of migraine. They studied 27 patients with migraine who were off medication during a headache-free period. The migraineurs showed a significantly lower ($p < 0.002$) circulating microemboli index (CMI) and a higher aggregation response to adenosine diphosphate (ADP) ($p < 0.025$) when compared with 35 normals.

Platelet function tests were performed in 14 migraine patients during the headache-free period and repeated subsequently in 11 patients during the prodrome and in 11 patients during the headache phase. Platelet adhesiveness to glass beads and aggregation response to ADP, epinephrine, thrombin and serotonin increased during the prodrome. During the headache phase, however, adhesiveness increased significantly ($p < 0.01$) and aggregation in response to ADP and epinephrine decreased significantly ($p < 0.0$ and $p < 0.05$).

The increase in platelet aggregation during the prodrome and decrease during the headache phase parallel the reported increase in plasma serotonin level during the prodrome and subsequent decrease during the headache phase. Since platelets contain all the serotonin present in blood and release it during aggregation, it is possible that changes in plasma serotonin levels in migraine are secondary to changes in platelet aggregation.

Sandler (1975) observed a platelet monoamine oxidase deficiency in migraine. He noted that a transitory but highly significant decrease in platelet monoamine oxidase activity was seen during headache attacks in migrainous subjects and reverted to normal during attack-free periods. This was not the result of drugs used for the treatment of migraine. It is possible that decreased platelet monoamine oxidase and 5-hydroxytryptamine occur in response to release into the circulation of an unidentified substance during the headache. Sandler draws attention to the biochemical relationship of migraine and depressive illness, an association well described in the past by others. (See Chapter 5.)

Local accumulation of a vasodilator polypeptide, akin to bradykinin, can be demonstrated in the subsurface tissues of patients with migraine (Chapman et al., 1960).

Tyramine, a pressor amine found in certain foods, can evoke migraine in susceptible subjects (Hanington, 1967). Tyramine liberates norepinephrine from tissues. A defect in the conjugation of tyramine has been reported in migraine patients, which has genetic implications since migraine is a familial if not a genetic disorder.

Temporal arteries removed from humans during the painful stage of migraine have an increased capacity to take up norepinephrine. Conversely, infusions of norepinephrine can be used to treat migraine.

The role of the complement cascade and immunoglobulin patterns in migraine remains controversial. Lord and Duckworth (1977) described significant alterations in serum complement components during headache and headache-free periods. However, more recent studies by Moore et al. (1980) failed to show any evidence of altered complement levels, of increased globulin levels, or of increased levels of immune complexes during migraine or headache-free periods. Moore et al. suggest that an immune complex mediated reaction does not participate in the platelet aggregation, serotonin release, and basophil and mast cell degranulation that have been associated with migraine headaches.

Prostaglandins have not been measured in humans with migraine, but injections of prostaglandins may produce headache in susceptible subjects (Peatfield et al., 1981).

In cluster headache, related to migraine, an increase in whole blood histamine levels has been demonstrated at the onset of an attack (Anthony and Lance, 1971). Injection of histamine and other vasodilators may provoke an attack in susceptible subjects with cluster headache.

MEDICATIONS

These observations and others have led to the therapeutic and prophylactic use of medications which inhibit the actions of some vasoactive substances, tend to stabilize membranes, reduce excessive vasomotor activity and interfere with the chemical mediators of inflammation (Fauchamps, 1975). Examples follow.

Medications are used to inhibit the actions of vasoactive substances, stabilize membranes and reduce vasomotor activity and inflammation.

Antihistamine and antiserotonin compounds will interfere with vasoactive amines or inhibit their elaboration from their respective depots.

Nonsteroidal anti-inflammatory drugs, including aspirin and indomethacin, stabilize proteins and inhibit the formation of active prostaglandins from their precursors. Aspirin reduces platelet aggregation and indirectly affects the release of vasoactive substances.

Corticosteroids reduce inflammation at several levels, lower the complement titer and stabilize lysosomal membranes. Experimental evidence indicates that corticosteroids

- inhibit release of histamine from mast cells, normalize capillary permeability and reduce exudation
- stabilize cell membranes, enhance cell resistance to cytotoxins and interrupt the chain reaction to cell breakage
- stabilize lysosome membranes
- stabilize capillaries and inhibit emigration of neutrophils (polymorphonuclear leukocytes)
- inhibit granulation, fibrosis and collagen deposition

Some anti-inflammatory drugs interfere with kinin functions or with the actions of prostaglandins.

Some drugs have multiple effects. Ergot, for example, is both a vasoconstrictor and an α-adrenergic blocker. Propranolol, a β-adrenergic blocker, is used in migraine prophylaxis. No single drug will block or inhibit all components of inflammation. Effective therapy may require the use of several.

The relationship between the efficacy of strictly antiserotonin compounds and migraine prophylaxis is a complex one. It seems evident with each passing year, however, that the specific antiserotonin activity of this or that compound has little to do with its efficacy in migraine. It simply is not enough to block the peripheral actions of serotonin alone and expect adequate migraine prophylaxis to be accomplished. Cyproheptadine, which blocks both serotonin and histamine, comes closest to this therapeutic situation. Methysergide, advertised as a serotonin antagonist, has complex pharmacologic effects. It also blocks histamine indirectly by interfering with histamine liberators, at least in vivo. Furthermore, as suspected early on, it has significant vasoconstrictor properties. Recent studies in the dog make it evident that methysergide produces profound vasoconstriction of the external carotid artery.

This being the case, the question may be posed regarding the etiologic role of the indolamine, serotonin, in the pathogenesis of migraine. The changes in the level of plasma serotonin observed prior to the onset of migraine may represent only one aspect of the genesis of migraine. Similarly, the importance of the changes of whole blood histamine prior to the onset of cluster headache is suspect. Other diseases in which there are great changes in blood histamine are not characterized by unilateral severe headache.

What seems more likely is that histamine, serotonin, the plasma kinins and perhaps other vasoactive substances participate in a sterile inflammatory reaction involving painful and distended blood vessels. They are, then, an integral but peripheral part of the migraine process and certainly one part of the process that can be measured and toward which therapy can be directed. But they are important primarily to that part of the migraine episode wherein *an increase in vascular permeability occurs.*

CENTRAL PROCESS OF MIGRAINE

This has been a brief summary of the peripheral aspects of migraine and the possible relationship of biochemical processes and vasoactive substances. Let us turn now for a moment to the central processes of migraine, for it is generally accepted that in classic migraine the intracranial vessels are profoundly affected. Indeed, it has been shown by cerebral blood flow measurements, utilizing radioactive gas as a marker, that the prodromes of migraine are associated with a profound reduction in blood flow to the cerebral cortex, sometimes focal, sometimes generalized.

Edmeads (1977) has described his study of cerebral blood flow in migraine. The results of these studies tend to confirm Wolff's hypothesis that cerebral blood flow is decreased during auras and increased during headaches. However, some findings were unexpected. The distribution in time and space of the blood flow changes did not always correlate with clinical features of the attack. Autoregulation of the cerebral blood vessels may be impaired in aura and in headache, and this is a key factor in intensifying and prolonging attacks.

The measurements of cerebral blood flow have made significant contributions to our knowledge of the pathogenesis of and effective therapy for migraine. In terms of practical therapeutics, Edmeads' study shows that ergotamine does not affect cerebral blood flow even when it has clearly been effective in ablating headache. This is an important observation, since the immunity of the intracranial circulation to ergotamine suggests that the traditional prohibition of this drug to patients who have severe vasoconstrictive auras may be unnecessary and that these patients may now receive the benefits of treatment at the onset of their aura, rather than waiting until the headache begins.

The theoretical implications of the blood flow studies are more far-reaching. They provide the additional evidence required to confirm Wolff's hypothesis regarding the vascular theory of migraine. Perhaps more important, these blood flow studies indicate that the Wolff theory, while correct, is also incomplete. The unexpected data on the frequent discrepancy between the spatial and temporal relationship of blood flow and the distribution of symptoms and the data on the disordered cerebral vasoreactivity during attacks will serve as points for further research into the mechanisms of migraine and the autonomic nervous system.

Welch et al. (1976) made biochemical comparisons between migraine and stroke. They measured γ-aminobutyric acid (GABA) and 3′,5′-cyclic adenosine monophosphate (cAMP) in the CSF of patients with stroke and vascular headache of migraine type. GABA was elevated in the CSF of patients with recent onset of thromboembolic occlusive cerebrovascular disease (CVD) and within 48 hours of an attack of vertebrobasilar ischemia (VBI). Similarly, GABA was elevated in the CSF of all patients studied during a migraine attack but not in asymptomatic migraine patients or patients with muscle contraction (tension) headache. CSF cAMP was also elevated in patients with recent onset of thromboembolic occlusive CVD and in patients studied during or within 48 hours of a migraine attack.

Since the biochemical abnormalities reported herein were common to occlusive CVD and migraine headache, it seems probable that they are due to the ischemia associated with both conditions and possibly are related to the resultant disorder of cerebral energy metabolism.

In recent years, interest has again focused on the role of the autonomic nervous system in the maintenance of cerebral vascular tone and blood flow. It is recognized that minute changes in the level of carbon dioxide in the blood significantly affect cerebral blood flow. This carbon dioxide regulating effect is more important than either hypoxia or hypoglycemia. A sudden fall in systemic arterial blood pressure will also evoke vasodilation.

If all these variables are controlled, however, is it possible to alter cerebral blood flow through stimulation of the autonomic nervous system? There is an abundant network of autonomic nerves in contact with the basal and pial arteries of the brain. Electron microscopic studies have shown that these nerves terminate in contact with vascular smooth muscle. Stimulation of the cervical sympathetic nerves can, in animals, produce constriction of the carotid and vertebral arteries to the extent of affecting tissue perfusion. These arteries can be made to constrict by local application of catecholamines and these responses can be blocked by adrenolytic agents. After prolonged spasm, stores of norepinephrine in the perivascular nerves are reduced.

Control of Cerebral Blood Flow

Olesen (1972) proposes a useful hypothesis for the control for cerebral blood flow, which has clinical implications with respect to migraine. He divides the cerebral blood vessels into two systems, dependent upon their adrenergic nervous supply. One system comprises the large arteries at the base of the brain and the pial arteries and is distinguished by its rich nerve supply and the responsiveness of the vessels to catecholamines (catecholamine responses can be blocked). The term "innervated vascular system" is suggested for these vessels. The other system, consisting of parenchymal vessels, has little or no autonomic innervation and responds only to the metabolic needs of the brain tissues to which it is closely approximated. These vessels are not responsive to application of catecholamines. The two systems of blood vessels are connected in series.

The character of the two systems relates structure to function. The blood vessels of the noninnervated system, being in close contact with brain tissues and regulated by their local metabolic needs, include the terminal high resistance arterioles. The innervated system, with its abundant nerve supply, regulates flow through the large arteries and is capable of reacting to external or nonlocal factors, thus protecting the parenchymal arteries in the brain from sudden increases or decreases in arterial pressure—for example, during active exercise. The dual system also allows maximum tissue blood flow if the systemic arterial blood pressure falls suddenly.

We suggest that, in migraine, the sudden neurogenic vasoconstriction of the great arteries of one internal carotid would lead to a temporary reduction in flow through the noninnervated system. The local metabolic demands of the brain would rapidly thereafter produce a focal acidosis and intracranial vasodilation, particularly of the noninnervated system but also involving the innervated system, which might be mirrored in the extracranial subsurface scalp tissues and so produce the typical hemicranial headache.

There is also some indirect evidence to support these concepts. Methysergide has peripheral and central effects and the central effects are at least in part mediated through inhibition of central vasomotor responses. The concentration of brain serotonin is, in animals, intimately related to the functions of the central vasomotor centers. It has been proposed that the central vasomotor centers and the central autonomic nervous system perform a neuroregulatory role in the control of the vascular tone of the major blood vessels at the base of the brain.

Unified Theory of Migraine

Hence, a unified theory of migraine emerges—a neurogenic concept of migraine. Subsequent to some stress or nonspecific or specific stimulus, the series of nervous reflexes which initiate the migraine process occurs. The preheadache vasoconstrictor phenomenon represents neurogenic vasospasm of the innervated vascular system at the base of the brain and the pial arteries (Fig. 1.1). This vascular activity represents the initial vector of vascular reaction in migraine. The vasoconstriction produces a relative reduction in local cerebral blood flow, with the consequent local metabolic tissue abnormalities including acidosis and anoxia (Fig. 1.2). The noninnervated parenchymal arteries, responsive to local metabolic demands, next dilate and if vasodilation is sufficiently great the cranial arteries on the outside of the head also expand (Fig. 1.3). The alteration in tone of the extracranial arteries provokes the liberation of multiple local chemical and vasoactive substances as described above, producing edema, a lowering of pain threshold and, eventually, pounding headache (Fig. 1.4). Since the initial vasoconstrictor phase may be focal or unilateral, so also the subsequent headache may be hemicranial. A suggestion is therefore provided for the enigma of the hemicranial aspect of migraine. (See also Plate 14.2.)

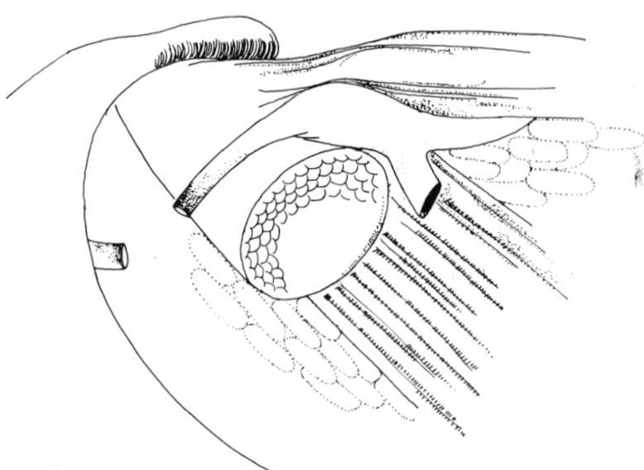

Figure 1.1. Clinical features of migraine vasoconstriction. The head pain is preceded by painless preheadache phenomena, particularly visual field defects. Other symptoms include speech difficulties, dizziness and weakness.

Furthermore, studies of the recently characterized endogenous opiates in migraineurs seem to indicate a physiologic inability to tolerate pain. CSF and plasma levels of the endogenous opiates are generally noted to rise during pain, a phenomenon which is thought to be crucial to pain modulation. Anselmi and others (1980) at the University of Florence measured levels of enkephalins, β-endorphin and tryptophan in migraine and cluster headache sufferers with the following results:

- decreased levels of CSF enkephalins in migraine attack and cluster headache

- increased serum β-endorphin-like immunoreactivity at the end of attack
- increased CSF and free plasma tryptophan in migraine

Thus, a dysfunctional central analgesia possibly predisposes such patients to recurrent

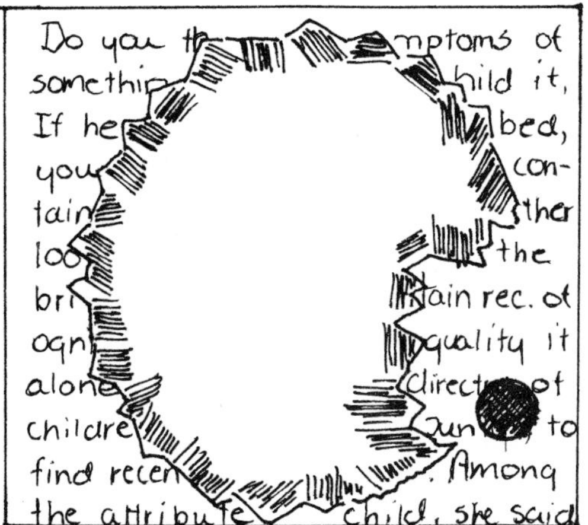

Figure 1.2. A typical migrainous field defect.

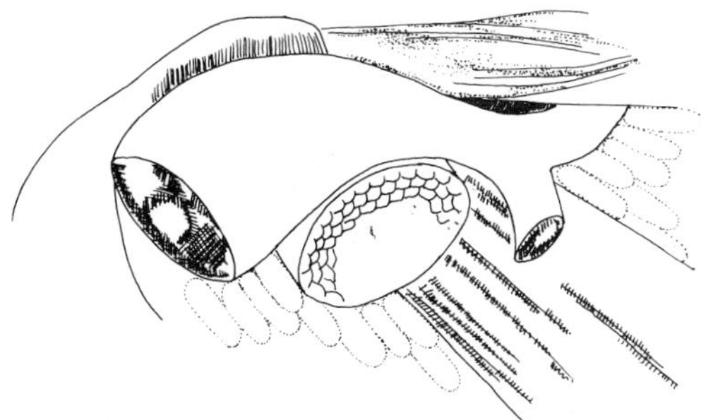

Figure 1.3. Vasodilation. Ordinarily there is one-sided throbbing pain associated with dilation of intracranial and extracranial blood vessels.

attacks. The observed increase in serum β-endorphin-like immunoreactivity may represent a response to headache-induced stress.

MUSCLE CONTRACTION HEADACHE

Muscle contraction (MC) headache ("tension headache") is characterized by an inability to relax the muscles of the scalp and neck. It is almost invariably associated with some form of depression, anxiety, psychosomatic illness or emotional conflict (Martin, 1966; Gainotti et al., 1970) and is frequently present in those afflicted by migraine. Serotonin has been implicated in MC headache as low CNS levels probably contribute to the pathogenesis of depression (Maas, 1975), while low blood levels have been found in MC headache sufferers when compared with normals and migraineurs (Rolf et al., 1977).

While the scalp vessels dilate in migraine attacks, the reverse occurs in MC headache.

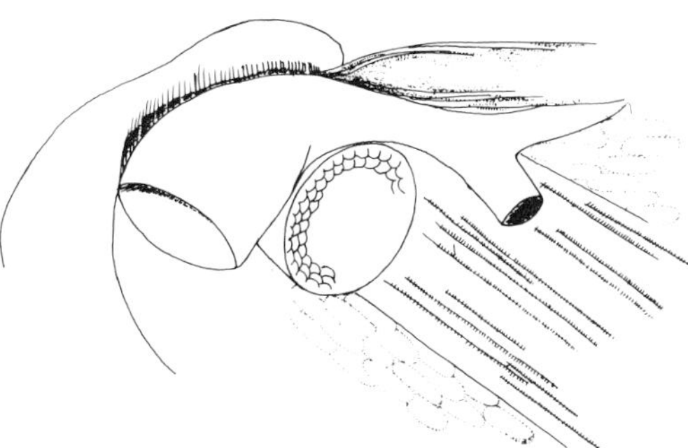

Figure 1.4. The edema phase. In this stage the headache becomes persistent and steady, associated with vascular edema, nausea, vomiting and general malaise.

The pain of MC headache worsens with vasoconstrictive drugs and is relieved by vasodilators; the small conjunctival vessels have been observed to constrict for the duration of the attack (Ostfeld et al., 1957).

Finally, MC headache sufferers may also be predisposed to recurrent pain by a dysfunctional central analgesia. The serotonin-containing neurons of the nucleus raphe magnus in the pons send axons which course through the lateral column of the spinal cord to synapse on endogenous opiate-containing neurons in the substania gelatinosa. The axons also terminate in similar neurons located in the spinal trigeminal nuclei (Fields, 1978 and 1981). Conceivably, a deficiency of serotonin could alter the normal response to pain. (See also Plate 14.4.)

SUMMARY

In summary, migraine can be viewed as a form of relatively benign vasospasm, usually unilateral. It is an episodic disorder produced by the interactions of the central and peripheral autonomic nervous systems, and the extracranial and intracranial blood vessels. It involves both central and peripheral vasomotor mechanisms, combined with a sterile inflammatory reaction, neurogenically induced.

Migraine can be viewed as a form of relatively benign vasospasm.

Muscle contraction itself does not completely explain MC headache. MC headache and the oft-associated clinical depression may be related to subnormal serotonin levels in the brain. The pain stems from tonic muscle contraction and vasoconstrictive muscle ischemia.

Migraineurs as well as MC headache patients may be abnormally subject to chronic pain as a result of deficient pain-modulating systems mediated by the endorphins and enkephalins.

References

Ad Hoc Committee (1962) Classification of headache. *JAMA 6:*717.

Anselmi B, Baldi E, Cassaci F, Salmon S (1980) Endogenous opioids in cerebrospinal fluid and blood in idiopathic headache sufferers. *Headache 20:*294–299.

Anthony M, Hinterberger H, Lance JW (1969) The possible relationship of serotonin to the migraine syndrome. *Res Clin Stud Headache 2:*29–59.

Anthony M, Lance JW (1971) Histamine and serotonin in cluster headache. *Arch Neurol 25:*225.

Basbaum AJ, Fields HL (1978) Endogenous pain control mechanisms: Review and hypothesis. *Ann Neurol 4:*451–462.

Chapman LF, Ramos AO, Goodell H, et al. (1960) Neurokinin: A polypeptide formed during neuronal activity in man. *Trans Am Neurol Assoc 85:*42

Deshmukh SV, Meyer JS (1977) Cyclic changes in platelet dynamics and the pathogenesis and prophylaxis of migraine. *Headache 17:*101–108.

Edmeads J (1977) Cerebral blood flow in migraine. *Headache 17:*148–152.

Fauchamps A (1975) Pharmacodynamic principles of antimigraine therapy. *Headache 15:*79–90.

Fields HL (1981) Pain: II. New approaches to management. *Ann Neurol 9:*101–106.

Gainotti G, Cianchetti C, Taramelli M (1970) Anxiety level and psychodynamic mechanisms in medical headaches: Psychodiagnostic study. *Res Clin Stud Headache 3:*182–190.

Hanington E (1967) Preliminary report on tyramine headache. *Br Med J 2:*550.

Lord GDA, Duckworth JW (1977) Immunoglobulin and complement studies in migraine. *Headache 17:*163.

Maas JW (1975) Biogenic amines and depression: Biochemical and pharmacological separation of two types of depression. *Arch Gen Psychiatry 32:*1357–1361.

Martin MJ (1966) Tension headache: A psychiatric study. *Headache 6:*47–54.

Moore TL, Ryan RE, Jr, Pohl DA, et al. (1980) Immunoglobulin, complement, and immune complex levels during a migraine attack. *Headache 20:*9–12.

Movat HZ (1972) Chemical mediators of the vascular phenomena of the acute inflammatory reaction and of immediate hypersensitivity. *Med Clin North Am 56:*541–546.

Müller-Eberhard HJ (1977) Chemistry and function of the complement system. *Hosp Pract 12:*33–43.

Olesen J (1972) The effect of intracarotid epinephrine, norepinephrine, and angiotensin on the regional cerebral blood flow in man. *Neurology 22:*978.

Ostfeld AM, Reis DJ, Wolff HG (1957) Studies on headache: Bulbar conjunctival ischaemia and muscle contraction headache. *Arch Neurol Psychiatry 77:* 113.

Peatfield RC, Gawel MJ, Rose FC (1981) The effect of infused prostacyclin in migraine and cluster headache. *Headache 21:* 190–195.

Ray BS, Wolff HG (1940) Experimental studies on headache: Pain-sensitive structures of the head and their significance in headache. *Arch Surg 41:*813.

Rolf LH, Wiele G, Brune GG (1977) Serotonin in platelets of patients with migraine and muscle contraction headache. *Excerpta Med 427:*11–12.

Sandler M (1975) Monoamines and migraine: A path through the woods. In *Vasoactive Substances Relevant to Migraine*, edited by Diamond S, et al. Springfield, IL, Charles C Thomas, pp. 3–18.

Sicuteri F (1967) Vasoneuroreactive substances and their implication in vascular pain. *Res Clin Stud Headache 1:*6–45.

Welch KMA, Chabi E, Nell JH, et al. (1976) Biochemical comparison of migraine and stroke. *Headache 16:*160–167.

2

Taking a Headache History

A detailed and relevant history geared to the headache patient is the most important factor in making correct diagnosis. By carefully questioning and directing the inquiry, a specific headache profile evolves which makes the diagnosis in many instances, for the majority of patients with headache have negative neurologic and physical examinations. The essentials of a headache history should be set down in a short, concise manner so that a pattern will evolve and the clinician will be able to identify the kinds of headache that are present.

Headache outlines at the end of this chapter depict the form used for the headache history. We start the headache history by asking the patient for a precise description of headache; it is quite common for a patient to have two or three separate types of headache. The charting of the headache frequency by the patient for 1 or 2 months (the headache calendar) often gives clues to the type of headache present. Table 2.1 shows a headache calendar kept by a migraine patient; Table 2.2 depicts migraine with depression.

Onset

We are interested in the specific time of life when the headaches began. Headaches that start in childhood, in adolescence and in the second and third decades of life are often vascular in nature, such as migraine. Headaches which occur later in life suggest an organic etiology or may be due to psychogenic ills such as depression. The occurrence of a headache after a traumatic episode, such as the death of a loved one, a serious financial loss, etc., may be a key to an underlying depression. Headaches due to high blood pressure are usually present on awakening and often disappear as the day goes on. Migraine can awaken a patient at 3 or 4 o'clock in the morning but, more often, cluster headaches occur at night and frequently awaken the patient several hours after going to sleep. Sinus headache usually begins gradually in the morning and increases in severity during the day. Headache related to anxiety without an obvious depressive component often follows a specific stressful incident (for example, the patient whose headache starts with the death of a brother from a brain tumor). Under the general heading of *onset* we also ask about the length of illness. Many migraine or depressive sufferers will give a 20-, 30- or 40-year history of the headache. The chronicity of their headache suggests that we are not dealing with a progressive neurologic lesion. Conversely, the sudden onset of severe headache and diagnostic neurologic signs precludes a self-limited headache syndrome.

LOCATION

It is important to know whether the cephalalgia is generalized over the entire head or whether it is localized on one side. It is also important to know whether the pain switches from one side of the head to the other, for migraine frequently acts in this way. Generalized head pain may indicate psychogenic disease, in the absence of increased intracranial pressure. Focal pain on one side of the head may be migraine but can also be due to organic disease. Pain localized to the eye alone should make one suspicious of either ocular disease or cluster headache. The "hatband" distribution of head pain speaks for muscle contraction headache.

FREQUENCY

Migraine may occur at sporadic intervals during a lifetime. By the time medical advice is

Table 2.1 Headache Calendar

Patient's Name:
Date Started: Oct. 13, 1972

DATE	TIME ONSET (Insert hr. and am/pm)	TIME ENDING (Insert hr. and am/pm)	(*1) SEVERITY OF HEADACHE	(*2) RELIEF OF HEADACHE	MEDICATION TAKEN AND DOSAGE	(*3) PSYCHIC AND PHYSICAL FACTORS	(*4) FOOD AND DRINK EXCESSES
10-13							
10-14	12:00 noon	4P	8	3	Cafergot - 2	#19	
10-15							
10-16							
10-17							
10-18							
10-19							
10-20							
10-21	10A	12N	6	3	Cafergot 1		J
10-22							
10-23							
10-24							
10-25							
10-26							
10-27							
10-28							
10-29							
10-30							
10-31							
11-1							
11-2	2P	3P	3	2	Cafergot 1	#15	
11-3							
11-4	4P	7P	7	5	Cafergot 3	#15	L
11-5							
11-6							
11-7							
11-8							
11-9							

Table 2.2 Headache Calendar

Patient's Name:
Date Started: Dec. 30, 1972

DATE	TIME ONSET (Insert hr. and am/pm)	TIME ENDING (Insert hr. and am/pm)	(*1) SEVERITY OF HEADACHE	(*2) RELIEF OF HEADACHE	MEDICATION TAKEN AND DOSAGE	(*3) PSYCHIC AND PHYSICAL FACTORS	(*4) FOOD AND DRINK EXCESSES
12/30/72	7AM	11A	5	4	Fiorinal x 2	10	
	2P	8P	6	4	Fiorinal x 2	10	
12/31/72	6P	12AM	8	3	Fiorinal x 4		M, S
1/1/73	10AM	3P	9	5	Fiorinal x 4	17	
1/2/73	11AM	8P	9	4	Fiorinal x 2	1	
1/3/73	8P	1A	9	5	Fiorinal x 3		N
1/4/73	8AM	11A	4	3	Fiorinal x 1	8	
1/5/73	6PM	10P	10	10	Fiorinal x 4	11	
					Cafergot x 2		
1/6/73	11P	1A	5	3	Fiorinal x 3	12	
1/7/73	8A	11A	4	4	Fiorinal x 2		C
	4P	9P	6	8	Fiorinal x 2	1	C
1/8/73	8A	11P	8	4	Fiorinal x 4	1	
1/9/73	8P	12A	5	3	Fiorinal x 4	6	S
1/10/73	10A	4P	4	3	Fiorinal x 2	17	
1/11/73	9A	11A	6	4	Fiorinal x 3	2	
1/12/73	6P	8P	2	1	Fiorinal x 1	7	
1/13/73	8A	7P	10	10	Fiorinal x 4	15	
					Cafergot x 3		
1/14/73	9A	5P	9	8	Fiorinal x 4	15	
1/15/73	9A	1P	6	4	Fiorinal x 2	15	
1/16/73	8P	12A	9	7	Fiorinal x 3	15, 1	
1/17/73	8A	11A	5	3	Fiorinal x 2	6	U
1/18/73	6P	9P	6	4	Fiorinal x 3	17	
1/19/73	8A	1P	8	7	Fiorinal x 3		
					Cafergot x 1	1, 18	
1/20/73	4P	9P	10	10	Fiorinal x 4	1	S
1/21/73	8A	11A	4	3	Fiorinal x 2		F
1/22/73	1P	3P	3	2	Fiorinal x 1	18	
1/23/73	8A	2P	7	6	Fiorinal x 4	6, 18	
1/24/73	4P	6P	3	2	Fiorinal x 1		G
1/25/73	10A	5P	6	5	Fiorinal x 3	10	

Headache Keys for Tables 2-1 & 2-2

HEADACHE KEYS

(*1) SEVERITY SCALE

1---+---+---+---5--+--+--+--+---10

None Mild Moderate Severe

(*2) RELIEF SCALE

1---+---+---+---5--+--+--+--+---10

Complete Moderate Mild No Relief

(*3) PSYCHIC & PHYSICAL FACTORS

1 - Emotional Upset/Family or Friends
2 - Emotional Upset/Occupation
3 - Business/Reversal
4 - Business/Success
5 - Vacation Days
6 - Weekends
7 - Strenuous Exercise
8 - Strenuous Labor
9 - High Altitude Location
10 - Anticipation Anxiety
11 - Crisis/Serious
12 - Post-Crisis Period
13 - New Job/Position
14 - New Move
15 - Menstrual Days
16 - Physical Illness
17 - Over-sleeping
18 - Weather
19 - Other ______________

(*4) FOOD & DRINK EXCESSES

A - Ripened Cheeses (Pizza)
B - Herring
C - Chocolate
D - Vinegar
E - Fermented Foods (pickled or marinated) (sour cream/yogurt)
F - Freshly Baked Yeast Products
G - Nuts (Peanut Butter)
H - Monosodium Glutamate (Chinese Foods)
I - Pods of Broad Beans
J - Onions
K - Canned Figs
L - Citrus Foods
M - Bananas
N - Pork
O - Caffeinated Bev. (Colas)
P - Avocado
Q - Fermented Sausage (Cured Cold Cuts)
R - Chicken Livers
S - Wine
T - Alcohol
U - Beer

sought, an identifiable pattern is often established. Commonly, in women there is an association with the menstrual cycle. Often there is an absence of the headache pattern during vacations and after the third month of pregnancy, but some headaches appear only during periods of relaxation. Cluster headache may be seasonal and often occurs in the spring and fall in bouts lasting from 1 to 2 weeks to 4 or 5 months. Rarely, cluster headache is chronic. The character of muscle contraction headache is one of chronicity and lasts for years, or a lifetime.

DURATION

If the headache is due to organic causes, it is usually continuous and progressively increases in intensity. The headache due to migraine is episodic and lasts anywhere from 6 hours to 3 days or even longer. Cluster head pain can last anywhere from several minutes to less than 4 hours. As mentioned above, muscle contraction headache is often persistent.

SEVERITY

The severity of the pain in migraine is often described as intense. Characteristically, it is pulsating or throbbing, rather than a constant pain. The pain of cluster headache is also throbbing, but it is frequently described as deep, boring and very severe. Tic douloureux is a shocklike, transient, stabbing pain, typically neuritic in character. Pain of muscle contraction headache is often dull, nagging and persistent, with occasional exacerbations of more severe pain.

The warning signs of migraine are usually ocular in nature.

PRODROMATA

Prodromata, or warning signs, are most common with migraine and are usually limited to visual symptoms (Table 2.3). It is believed that both the positive and negative eye prodromes originate in the visual cortex portion of the occipital lobe. The metamorphopsias indicate a disturbance of function in the optic radiation of the posterior temporal zone. Other aura may take the form of paresthesias, defects in mobility and, rarely, a disturbance of the sense of smell. Tumors and angiomas of the occipital lobe can also cause teichopsia, or fortification spectra, but they occur more persistently than in migraine.

ASSOCIATED SYMPTOMS

The migraine attack may include a wide variety of symptoms occurring in association with the pain. Photophobia, nausea, vomiting and urinary and focal neurologic changes may be seen. With cluster headache, a modified Horner's syndrome may appear, including ptosis and constriction of the pupil (Fig. 2.1). Lacrimation, flushing or blanching of the face and a mucoid discharge from the nostril on the side of the headache are often present with the cluster headache. Overt glaucoma is characterized by a steamy cornea and difficulty in seeing (Fig. 2.2). If subarachnoid hemorrhage has occurred, meningeal signs will appear rapidly. Sudden loss of power in the arms or legs with associated headache suggests a stroke, either thrombotic or hemorrhagic. Be alert to unilateral tinnitus or diplopia, which may be evidence of an intracranial mass. Associated epilepsy is usually an ominous sign.

SLEEP HABITS

Difficulty in falling asleep is indicative of anxiety. The doctor should look for an environmental stress syndrome or for psychologic factors which may be producing the problem. If the patient has frequent and early awakening, depression is suggested and questioning should be directed toward a possible depressive illness. Migraine patients can be awakened by severe headache during the night but are usually helped by sleep. Cluster headache patients are frequently awakened by their severe head pain, and the intensity of the pain forces them into ceaseless activity until the attack subsides.

PRECIPITATING FACTORS

Among the multiple factors which precipitate migraine are fatigue, loss of sleep, stress, menstruation, bright sunlight and foods and drugs containing tyramine and other vasoactive materials. Less common factors include alcohol, prolonged hunger and high humidity. Cough headache, contrary to popular belief, is not always associated with an intracranial tumor, can often be benign and may occur as a part of a vascular headache syndrome.

EMOTIONAL FACTORS

The patient's relationship to his/her family, occupation, social life, environmental stresses and sexual habits should all be ascertained in detail by the interviewer. Emotional factors such as these have special relevance to headache. Careful questioning about other physical, emotional and psychic symptoms may uncover an underlying psychologic illness that has been masked by the cephalalgic patient. Overt depression will be obvious to the interviewer. It is possible to uncover a stressful situation with associated anxiety by doing a simple inventory of the factors mentioned above.

RELATIONSHIP TO OCCUPATION

Emotional factors and stress on the job are common headache causatives. There are certain specific occupations, however, that have a built-in predisposition to head pain. Those dealing with the public in the provision of services are particularly susceptible. Abattoir workers are subject to Q fever, with intense headache as one of the symptoms. The nitrites to which munitions workers are exposed cause vasodilatation of the cerebral vessels and mimic vascular headaches. Mechanics and others can get headaches from the carbon monoxide in poorly ventilated work areas.

Some environmental exposures will cause headaches.

FAMILY HISTORY

Migraine is a familial illness, while cluster headache is not. Depression also is frequent in families. Studies suggest a hereditary relationship of migraine. If both parents have had migraine, there is a 70% chance that the children will also have migraine; if only one parent has had migraine, the chances are reduced to about 45%. If neither parent has had migraine but there is a history of migraine in other family members, it will occur in perhaps 25% of the children.

SEASONAL RELATIONSHIP

Cluster headaches are more common in the spring and fall. Depression with chronic headache often occurs during happy periods of the year, such as Christmas.

MENSTRUAL AND OBSTETRIC FACTORS

A common type of migraine occurs with the onset of menses. It tends to disappear by the third month of pregnancy only to return after the birth of the child. Migraine in women often disappears with onset of menopause. The administration of hormones in the postmenopausal period can prolong the headache syndrome. Conversely, migraine which reappears at the time of the menopause may be relieved by ingestion of estrogens.

In view of the increasing incidence of hyperprolactinemia, every female patient should be specifically questioned about the presence of galactorrhea and amenorrhea.

Table 2.3 Ocular Prodromata of Migraine

Positive	Teichopsia, or fortification spectra Zig zags Flashing lights and colors
Negative	Scotomata Hemianopsia
Metamorphopsia	Illusions of distorted size, shape and location of fixed objects

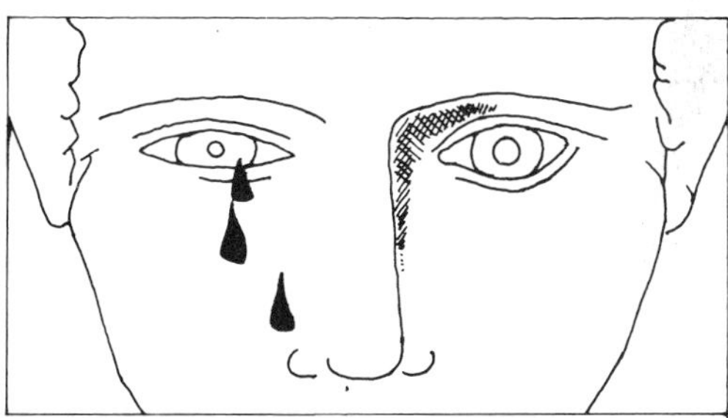

Figure 2.1. Horner syndrome and cluster headache: enophthalmos, ptosis of the eyelid, myosis of the pupil, lacrimation.

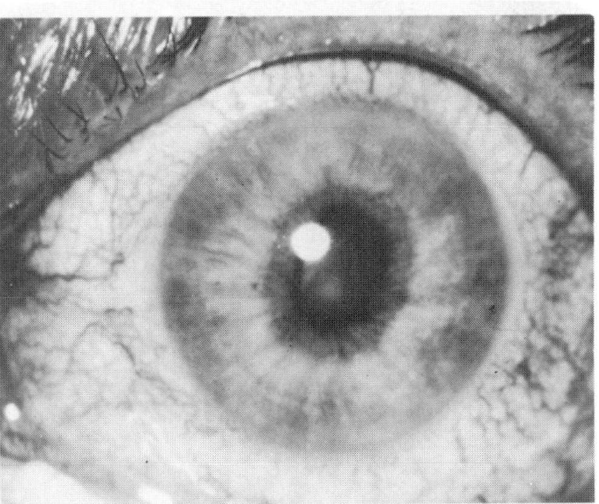

Figure 2.2. Steamy cornea indicates overt glaucoma.

MEDICAL HISTORY

Questions should also be asked regarding recent or remote head trauma. Subdural hematomas may occur after trivial blows. A recent spinal tap done for reasons of anesthesia or diagnosis may cause a self-limited headache. A low spinal fluid pressure syndrome has been described, which can be associated with a chronic subdural hematoma. A history of seizures, one-sided headache and neck stiffness should make one question whether there is an aneurysm or angioma present with a slow leak.

SURGICAL HISTORY

If a person has had surgery on a mole or other tumor it may follow that the tumor has metastasized to the brain, producing headache (Fig. 2.3). A past history of tuberculosis may have significance as to possible spread to the brain. Obviously, any previous cranial surgery will alert the physician to previous head trauma, tumor, aneurysm or other significant brain disease.

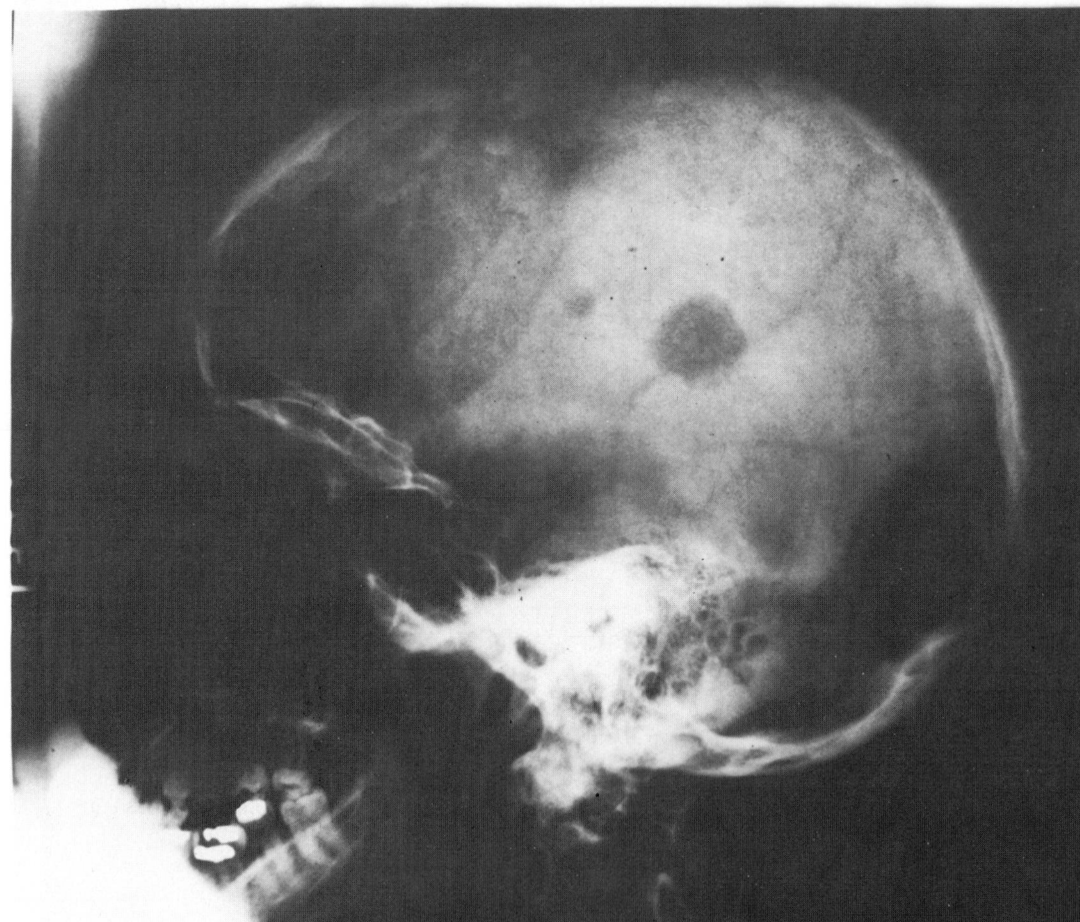

Figure 2.3. Multiple lucencies in a patient with previous carcinoma of the breast complaining of nonspecific headache.

SYSTEMS REVIEW

A complete, careful review of the systems should be done in all headache workups.

tinues to consume rather large amounts of aspirin regularly.

Headache 3 Outline

Types	One
Onset	At age 39
Location	Pain about forehead; occasional pain in cervical spine and occiput
Frequency	Almost daily
Duration	Constant
Severity	Severe
Aura	None
Associated symptoms	None
Emotional status	Feels unwell, irritable, nervous and depressed
Sleep pattern	Problems getting to sleep; often has early awakening
Family history	None
Seasonal	Not related

Headache 4: Cluster (Fig. 2.7)

R. B., aged 45, is a successful contractor who has always enjoyed good health. He was a former athlete but in recent years has exercised little and has gained 30 pounds in the last decade. He smokes heavily and on occasion drinks to excess. About 2 years ago he had a series of excruciating, usually nocturnal headaches, which began suddenly, lasted 3 weeks, and then ceased spontaneously. His physician was contacted at that time but offered no explanation for these episodes.

One month ago the nocturnal headaches began again. They often waken him at 3 AM and are localized to and above the left eye. The left eye waters copiously with the onset of headache. The left side of the nose is plugged initially and then runs later. His left eye becomes very red, perhaps because he rubs it. The pain is steady and intense, severe enough to make this stolid man cry for help. The pain usually lasts 45 mintues then rapidly clears; thereafter, he feels perfectly well. He has noticed, however, that even small amounts of alcohol can reproduce this set of symptoms and so he has stopped drinking completely in the last month. His physician was contacted again and advised R. B. that he was working too hard and was too tense. He went away for a week's vacation but the headaches continued. He began to worry that he might have a brain tumor. In the last several days, however, the headaches have again begun to disappear and are no longer so intense. He has not responded to any of several pain medications provided by his physician.

Headache 4 Outline

Types	One
Onset	Two years ago
Location	Above left eye
Frequency	Nightly
Duration	45 minutes
Severity	Severe
Aura	None
Associated symptoms	Left eye tears; nose stuffy
Allergy	None; alcohol brings on headache
Sleep pattern	Not affected
Emotional status	None
Family history	None
Seasonal	Spring and fall

Headache 5: Subarachnoid Hemorrhage (Fig. 2.8)

J. S., a 29-year-old man, was in his usual state of good health. He maintained his weight at moderate levels and practiced abstemious habits. A recent complete physical examination had been within normal limits. He had never complained of headache. Two weeks ago, while jogging, he experienced a sudden and severe head pain involving his entire head; the pain did not wax and wane and was not relieved by rest. He became ill and vomited and found no relief from aspirin, codeine or an ice pack applied to his head by his wife. Shortly thereafter he became sleepy and was not easily roused. His wife recognized immediately that a serious illness had occurred and she brought him to the emergency room of a hospital close by, but he could not walk from the car to the examining room. On admission he was restless and moaning in pain and could not give an adequate history. One pupil had become dilated but other signs of neurologic damage were not prominent. He was not paralyzed. He had developed slight stiffness of the neck. Computed tomography (CT) scan of the head demonstrated blood in the ventricular system. A spinal tap was done within the hour and the spinal fluid obtained was bloody. After consultation among several specialists, angiograms were done which showed a leaking aneurysm of one of the brain arteries. This was eventually clipped successfully by a neurosurgeon and J.S. is now recovering rapidly.

Aura	None
Associated symptoms	Vomiting, gradually became drowsy and comatose, dilation of one pupil, slight stiffness of the neck
Sleep pattern	Not affected
Emotional status	None related
Family history	None with headaches

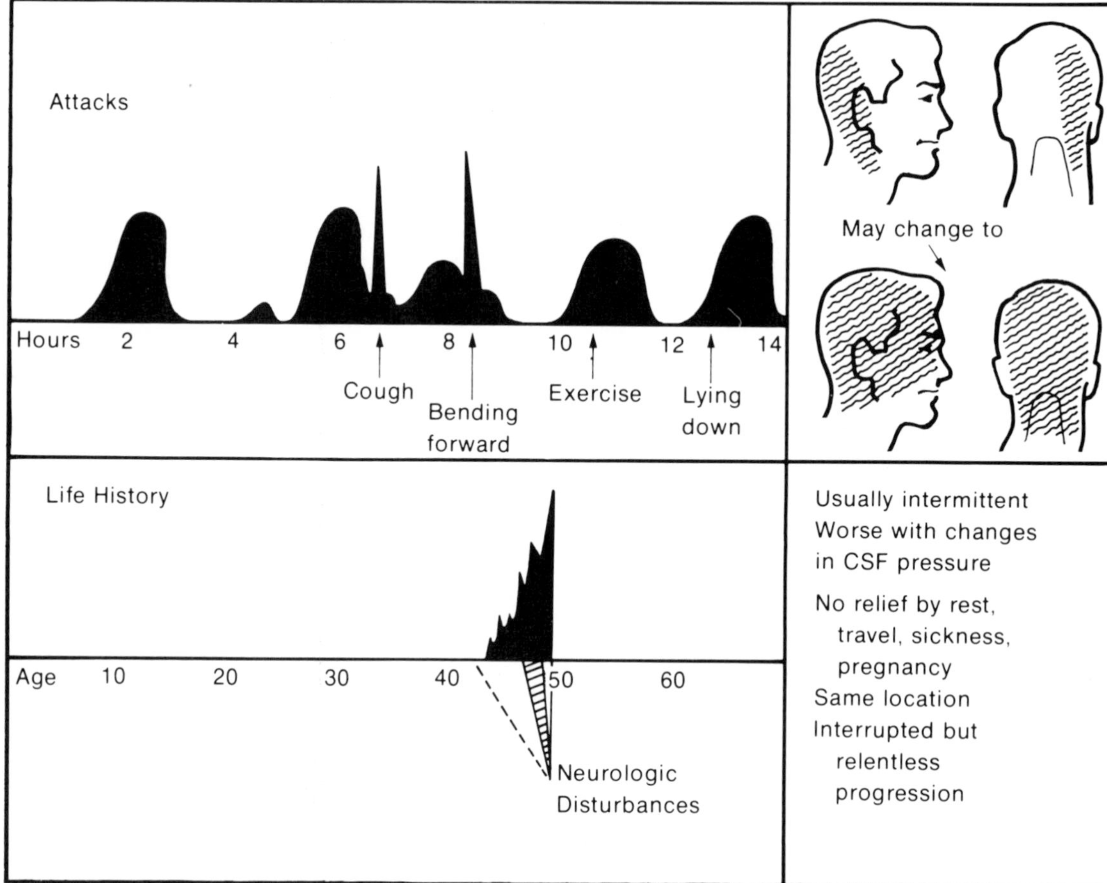

Figure 2.8. Aneurysm and angioma. (Adapted with permission of Graham J: Seven common headache profiles. Neurology 13:16–23, 1963. Copyright New York Times Media Company.)

Headache 5 Outline

Types	One
Onset	Age 29; 2 weeks prior to first visit
Location	Entire head; occurred while jogging
Frequency	One—the initial attack
Duration	Constant and unrelenting
Severity	Severe
Seasonal	Not related
Medical history	Negative
Surgical history	Negative
Allergy	None to medications or food
Tests	No previous examinations done
Medications	Aspirin, codeine, no relief

Headache 6: Brain Tumor (Fig. 2.9)

L. R., aged 60, began to note difficulty with his vision. He stated that his vision to the right was impaired. He found it difficult to read. He was bumping into objects on the right side of his environment. He saw an ophthalmologist who performed visual fields and elicited a field defect, although the patient's cooperation was not optimal.

L. R. has a long history of chronic frontal and temporal headaches which he associates with hay fever and sinusitis. He says that this has not increased, but during the course of the interview and examination he later states that he has more pain in the left side of the head which is relatively constant and now not easily relieved by medications. He describes great turmoil recently associated with problems with the Internal Revenue Service. These business difficulties have been very trying and he blames many of his current complaints on them. He takes large amounts of medication, including a sleeping pill, a tranquilizer, and an antihistamine, and he uses cigarettes and alcohol liberally.

When examined, he had a significant loss of visual acuity with a definite visual field cut on the right. His recent memory was poor. His speech was slow and suggested sedation.

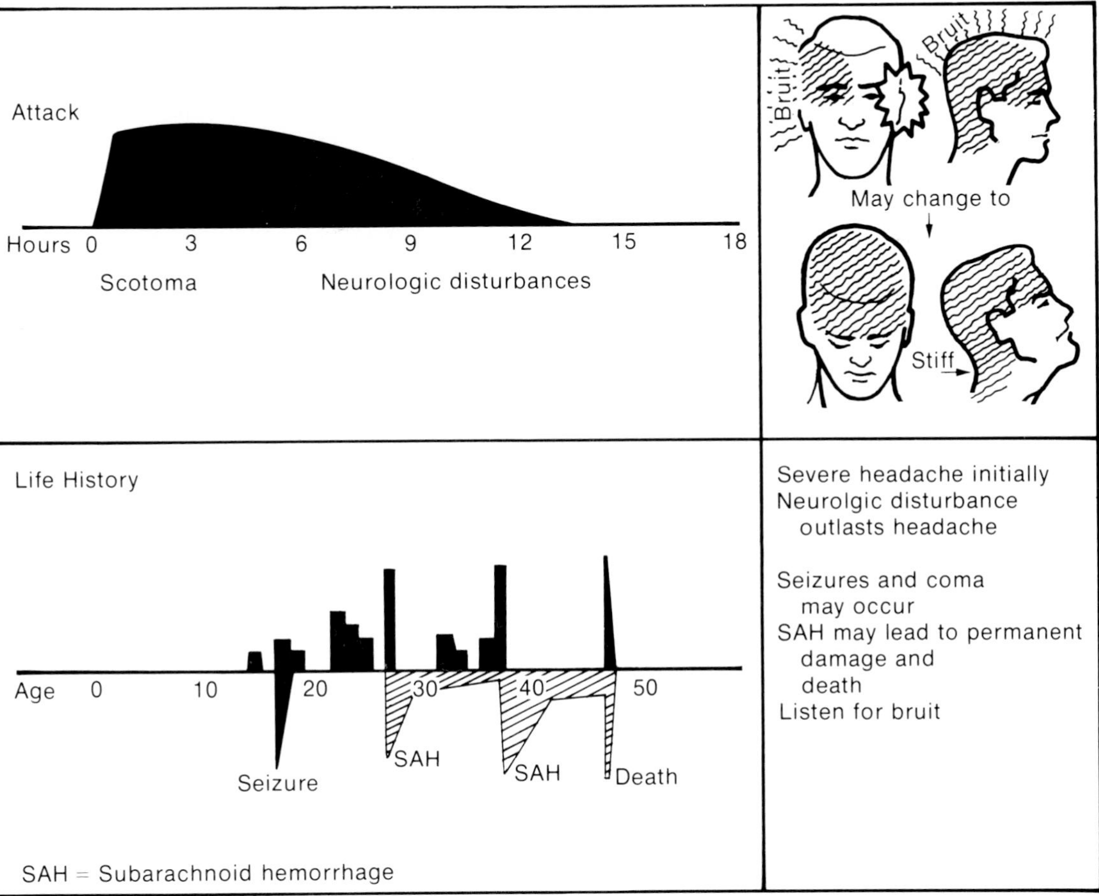

Figure 2.9. Brain tumor. (Adapted with permission of Graham J: Seven common headache profiles. Neurology 13:16–23, 1963. Copyright New York Times Media Company.)

There was minimal weakness of the right leg. The patient followed directions poorly and seemed confused.

He was admitted to a hospital where appropriate studies were done and a mass lesion was found in the left temporal and occipital area of the brain. He was transferred to a neurosurgical facility where a well-circumscribed and encapsulated tumor was removed. The patient has made an excellent recovery, is now free of headaches and is no longer confused, but still has a slight right visual field defect. He continues to complain of difficulties with the Internal Revenue Service.

Headache 6 Outline

Types	One
Onset	One year
Location	Frontal and temporal areas
Frequency	Constant
Duration	All day and night
Severity	Moderate to severe
Aura	None
Associated symptoms	Vision impaired; speech slowed; some confusion
Sleep pattern	Has trouble falling asleep
Emotional-status	Irritable
Family history	None
Seasonal	Not related

Headache 7: Brain Tumor

Mrs. W. T., aged 29, had complained for 2 months of "spin-outs," a sensation of unsteadiness and unreality associated with the feeling she might fall. She has had mild headaches in the left frontal area and above the left ear, but these have been relieved by aspirin until recently. Now, however, she notes an increase in headache, particularly when she coughs. She describes early morning nausea and loss of appetite. Her speech has slowed appreciably and has recently seemed slurred at times, and she sleeps often. She is forgetful. Her husband notes that her handwriting appears sloppy. He has also commented on intermittent twitching of the right side of her face and right hand. These complaints have progressed rapidly and inexorably.

When examined by her physician there were signs of increased pressure in the head, with weakness of the right arm and hand. She was admitted to a hospital where x-rays of the skull were done, which were normal, but the electroencephalogram and CT scan showed a mass lesion in the left frontal area of the brain. Operation was attempted, but the tumor which was found was too large to be removed. It did not respond to radiation therapy after surgery. Six months after the onset of symptoms, Mrs. W. T. was dead.

Headache 7 Outline

Types	One
Onset	Left frontal area—above left ear
Duration	All day
Frequency	Daily
Severity	Moderate to severe
Aura	None
Associated symptoms	Vertigo; nausea and loss of appetite; speech slurs; forgetful; handwriting sloppy; twitching of right face and head
Sleep pattern	Headache keeps her awake
Emotional status	Agitated since headaches started
Family history	None
Seasonal	Not related
Menses	Not related

Reference

Graham J (1963) Seven common headache profiles. *Neurology 13:*3, part 2, 16–23.

3

Physical and Neurological Examination of the Headache Patient

Every headache patient, after an all-inclusive history, deserves a complete physical and neurologic examination. Often there will be no significant findings, but this cannot be assumed, even if the medical history suggests a specific diagnosis. An outline of the examination covers

- general survey and physical examination
- mental state
- head
- cervical spine
- cerebellar functions
- cranial nerves
- motor functions
- sensory functions
- pathologic reflexes

GENERAL SURVEY AND PHYSICAL EXAMINATION

The facial characteristics and overall actions of a headache patient may give clues to the diagnosis. Depressed patients are frequently easy to spot by the down-turning of the corners of their mouths and their generally sad appearance (Fig. 3.1). The migraine patient may have her clothes neatly folded and will often fold her paper examination gown upon completion of the examination. Meticulous attention to personal appearance is a clue to the migrainous subject. Lists of symptoms and medications and careful documentation of headache frequency are other characteristics of the migraine patient (Fig. 3.2).

The cluster patient may, during an attack, exhibit a complete or partial Horner's syndrome with ptosis, a constricted pupil of the affected eye and flushing of the face; eye and nasal lacrimation may also occur. Graham

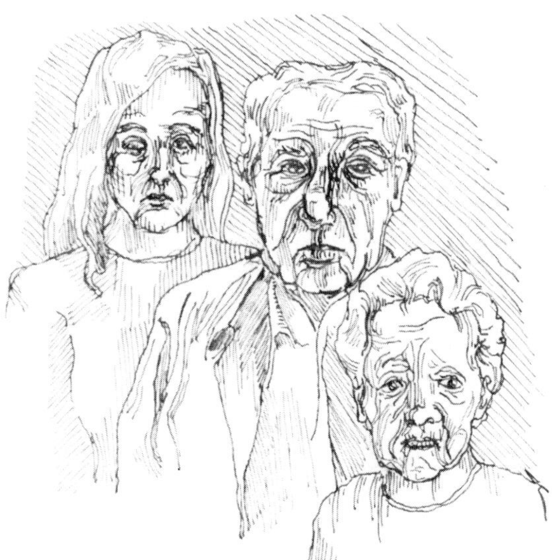

Figure 3.1. Depression.

(1974) has described the typical facial characteristics seen in a cluster patient: flushed appearance, square jaw, accentuated glabellar creases, thick chin and well-chiseled lower lip. Careful examination of the skin reveals telangiectases, coarse cheek skin (peau d'orange) and accentuated skin folds (Figs. 3.3 and 3.4).

Sometimes the diagnosis of facial pain is obvious, for example as in postherpetic neuralgia where there are trophic changes in the skin related to the antecedent viral infection (Fig. 3.5). Evidences of neurofibromatosis, with more than five accompanying brownish disk lesions of the skin (cafe-au-lait spots), may indicate an increased predilection for intracranial tumors, particularly neuromas and meningiomas (Fig. 3.6). Angiomata of the skin makes one suspicious of intracranial angioma. External evidences of hypothyroidism, including puffy, dry skin, brittle hair and loss of hair, can be associated with headache. We have seen several patients with hypothyroidism and bizarre chronic headache of an uncertain type. Pituitary deficiency with smooth skin, lack of body hair and testicular atrophy may also be an infrequent cause of chronic headache, if a pituitary tumor is present. Galactorrhea may be the sole manifestation of a prolactinoma.

One should question the headache patient carefully regarding surgical scars, since these can be a clue to cerebral metastases, especially from lesions such as melanomas.

The general physical examination may reveal many disparate illnesses which can cause headache. Hypertension, coarctation of the aorta and abnormalities of the cervical spine are but a few.

Patient is often a woman
Trimly built
Well dressed
Attractive
Answers questions quickly and to the point
Perfectionist—everything done on time and just so
Subject to fatigue

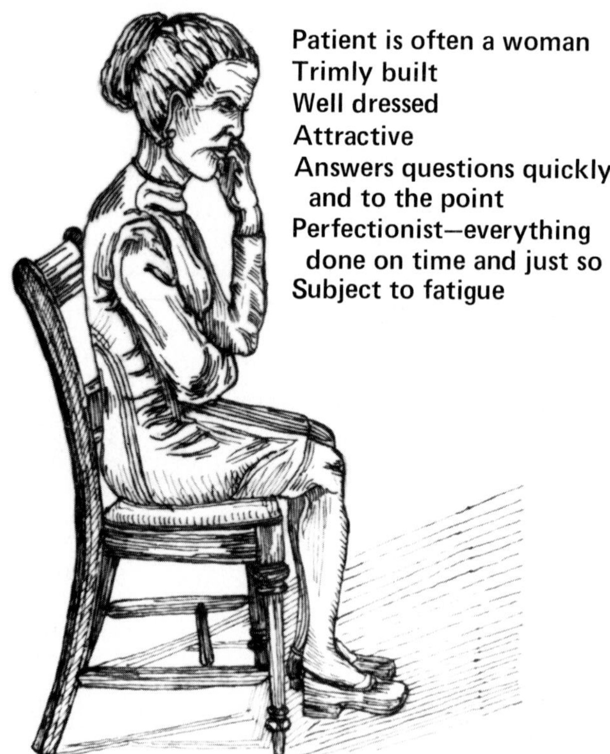

Figure 3.2. Frequent characteristics of migraine patients.

Physical examination may reveal many illnesses causing headache.

A distended bladder should be sought in the general physical examination of a patient with headache, since this can be a cause of reflex "autonomic headache." Although headache caused by distended bladder is most common in paraplegics, it can occur in others.

MENTAL STATE

This subject has been covered in part during the gathering of the history but can be further assessed during the physical examination. Examine orientation, memory, intelligence and speech. Obvious indications of either anxiety or depression may be present. Agitation and ceaseless activity may be evident. Failure to carry out the necessary tasks of the examination suggests inattention or dementia. Aphasia and other disorders of speech occurring in a right-handed person indicate a lesion of the left hemisphere. Memory impairment for recent events and failure to remember relevant details discussed only a few minutes before should alert the examiner to early dementia which, if accompanied by chronic headache, will require intensive neurologic investigation.

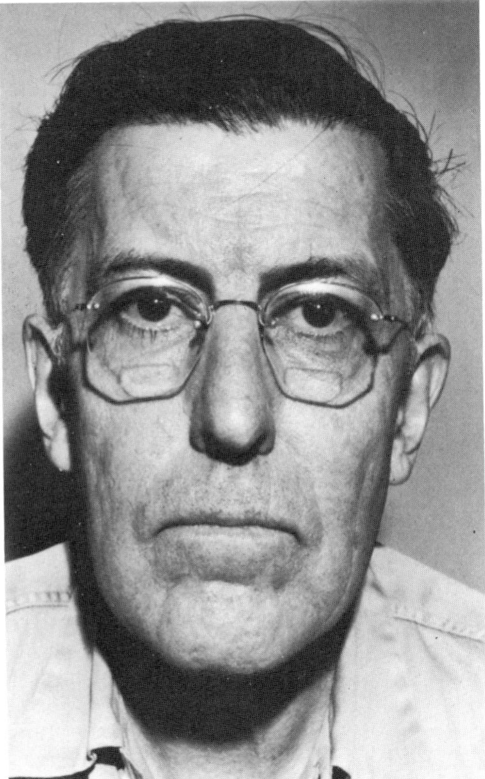

Figure 3.3. Patient exhibits typical facial characteristics of cluster headache.

HEAD

A careful examination of the head is required in all patients suffering cephalalgic pain. Evidence of local infection, hardened temporal arteries (temporal arteritis), a trigger point (tic douloureux), dysfunction of the temporal mandibular joint with spasm of muscles of mastication and crepitus, and tenderness over one of the sinus areas should be carefully sought in all patients. One should perform auscultation of the head and neck, searching for bruits which may be a clue to a possible aneurysm, carotid stenosis or angioma. Headache which occurs with coughing or with to-

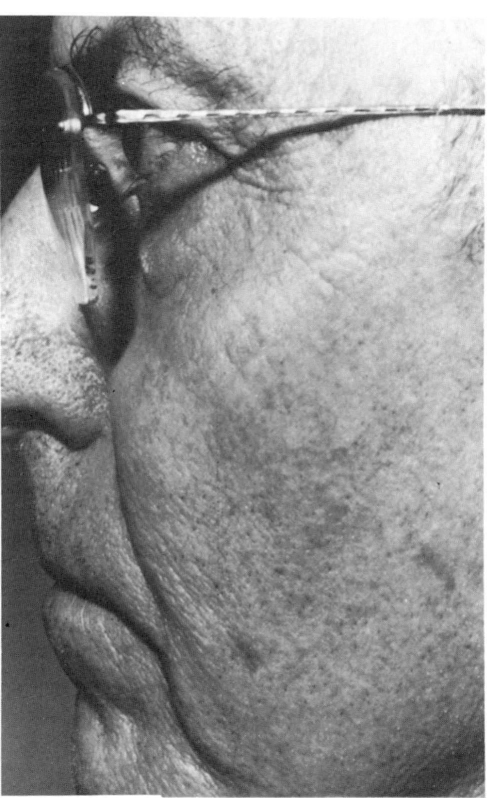

Figure 3.4. Closer examination of same patient reveals telangiectasis, peau d'orange and accentuated skin folds.

and-fro movements of the head may indicate a midline lesion, such as a cyst of the third ventricle.

CERVICAL SPINE

Muscle spasm, rigidity and reduced range of motion of the cervical spine can be indicative of muscle and/or spinal disease of the neck as a cause of chronic head and neck pain. Cervical spondylosis with headache is common in the elderly.

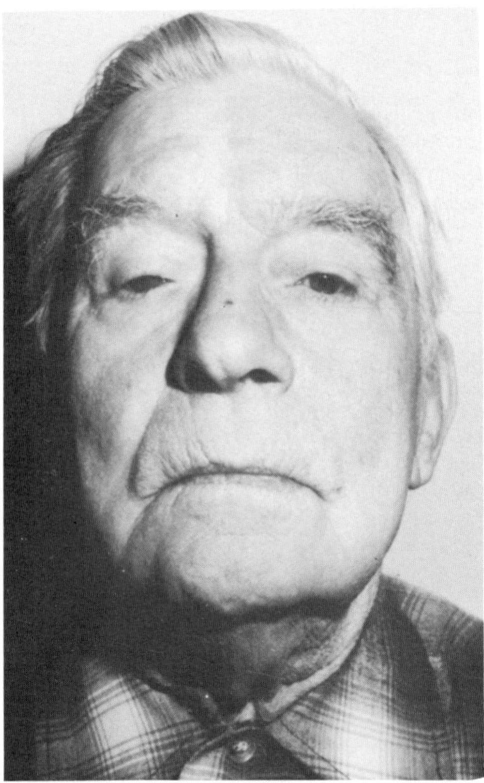

Figure 3.5. Postherpetic neuralgia.

CEREBELLAR FUNCTIONS

Cerebellar tumors, primary or metastatic, cerebellopontine angle tumors and large acoustic neuronomas may produce dyscoordination and signs of truncal ataxia with associated difficulties in equilibrium and steady movement. A wide-based gait is a common early manifestation of cerebellar disease. Abnormal finger-to-nose and/or heel-to-knee tests are often indications of cerebellar dysfunction. Headache is relatively uncommon in cerebellar disorders unless increased intracranial pressure develops.

CRANIAL NERVES

Olfactory Nerve (I)

Loss of sense of smell is most often due to local pathology in the nose and its accessory structures. A head injury or a tumor of the olfactory nerve in the olfactory groove may cause a unilateral disturbance of smell. If there is accompanying mental confusion, a frontotemporal tumor is suspected.

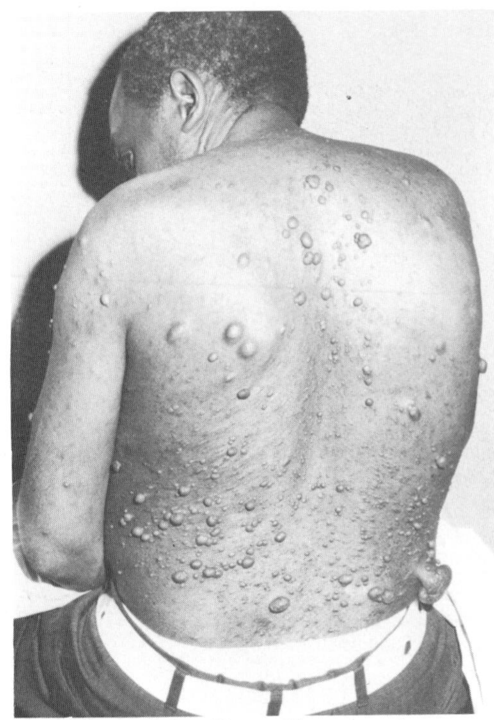

Figure 3.6. Neurofibromatosis.

Tests may indicate cranial nerve dysfunction causing headache.

Optic Nerve (II)

An eye examination is most important and must be included in the study of every headache patient. Simple observation may reveal the "steamed cornea" so typical of overt glaucoma. Testing of the pressure with the fingers can also elicit a difference in pressure between the two eyes. This should be confirmed with a tonometer. Gross examination of the visual fields should be performed and, if the exam is in any way abnormal, the visual fields should be plotted. Examination of the fundi is imperative since evidence of papilledema, optic atrophy, hemorrhages or exudates may indicate an organic brain lesion, hypertension or diabetes, among other diagnoses.

Abducens Nerve (VI)

Lesions, such as a lateral sinus thrombosis, may produce a unilateral sixth nerve paralysis. Bilateral sixth nerve paralyses may occur in acute hydrocephalus or cerebral edema.

Trigeminal Nerve (V)

The face and mucous membranes of the head should be examined for the trigger points of trigeminal neuralgia. Corneal testing should be performed with a wisp of cotton. Motor function of the trigeminal nerve is tested by opening the jaw against resistance.

Facial Nerve (VII)

This nerve is evaluated by testing the motor power of the facial muscles. Evidences of a residual stroke or facial palsy may be elicited.

Table 3.1. Clinical Manifestations of Temporal Lobe Herniation

Compressed Structure	Clinical Manifestations
Third cranial nerve	Dilated pupil ispsilateral to herniation
Midbrain	
Physiologic transection	Decerebrate rigidity
Reticular formation	Impairment of consciousness progressing to coma
Ipsilateral cerebral peduncle (direct compression)	Contralateral hemiparesis progressing to hemiplegia
Occlusion of aqueduct of Sylvius	Headache due to acute hydrocephalus
Contralateral cerebral peduncle (displaced against the sharp free edge of the tentorium)	Hemiparesis ipsilateral to herniation (false localizing sign)
Posterior cerebral artery as it crosses the tentorial edge to reach the occipital lobe (calcarine cortex)	Contralateral homonymous hemianopsia, false localizing sign

Oculomotor Nerve (III), Trochlear Nerve (IV)

A patient who complains of sudden pain behind the eye, with an accompanying third nerve palsy, should be evaluated for an expanding aneurysm. If the pupil on one side shows progressive enlargement, progressive compression of the oculomotor nerve is suggested. Herniation of the temporal lobe through the tentorium should be suspected (Table 3.1).

Remember that the upper part of the face is bilaterally innervated and that the lower part of the face is contralaterally innervated. There are four possible levels of facial nerve dysfunction on a peripheral basis, as follows, from above downward:

1. A lesion at or proximal to the geniculate ganglion will lead to loss of tearing of the ipsilateral eye, hyperacusis, paralysis of the facial muscles and loss of taste of the anterior two thirds of the tongue.

2. A lesion above the origin of the muscle to the stapedius gives rise to all of the findings mentioned above, but loss of tearing of the ipsilateral eye will not be noted.
3. Involving the facial nerve in the facial canal above the origin of the chorda tympani gives rise to the lesions mentioned above, excluding hyperacusis and loss of tearing of ipsilateral eye.
4. Involving the facial nerve at the stylomastoid foramen or below produces weakness of the facial muscles. Taste, hearing and tearing are unaffected.

With a suprasegmental facial paresis, the lower part of the face is more profoundly affected than the brow, since the brow is bilaterally innervated.

The face may also be affected in lesions of the basal ganglia as in Parkinson's disease. Here lack of movement of the face is primarily noted.

Auditory Nerve (VIII)

Both cochlear and vestibular functions should be tested. Simple tests of hearing should be done. Procedures such as calorics and rotational tests may be necessary. Unilateral tinnitus and deafness should always be investigated, to rule out an acoustic neuroma. Posterior fossa myelography and angiography may be necessary.

Glossopharyngeal, Vagus, Accessory and Hypoglossal Nerves (IX, X, XI, XII)

Most often involvement of these structures is not associated with serious headache problems. Lingual pain may occur in cranial arteritis. Bilateral absence of the pharyngeal reflex may be a hysteric phenomenon, but disease of the brainstem should also be ruled out.

MOTOR FUNCTIONS

Basically there are three motor systems. These include:

1. The pyramidal or corticospinal system. Lesions of this system produce paralysis or weakness, spasticity and hyperactive deep tendon reflexes.
2. Lesions of the extrapyramidal system produce instability of posture and disorders of muscle tone, as well as slowness of movement in nonparalyzed limbs.
3. The cerebellar system involves primarily accuracy of movements of the trunk and limbs. The cerebellum can be divided into two basic functional parts. The vermis is related to movements of the trunk, while the hemispheres serve especially coordination of the extremities, particularly the arms. It is also important to remember that the cerebellar tracts cross twice so that a lesion involving the right cerebellar hemisphere gives difficulty with the right arm and right leg.

Lower motor neuron disease is characterized by wasting, weakness, atrophy and loss of deep tendon reflexes, depending upon the extent of the lesion.

SENSORY FUNCTIONS

Central or peripheral lesions of the nervous system can be uncovered by careful sensory testing. Two-point discrimination is particularly important in assessing cortical sensation. A disturbance of astereognosis, or failure to recognize the size or shape of objects, can be the only sign of a parietal lobe tumor.

Remember that the basic sensory pathway consists of a three-neuron pattern. The primary sensory neuron has its cell body outside the central nervous system, usually in the dorsal root ganglia. The second neuron must cross the midline. The third neuron must have its cell body in the opposite thalamus and radiates thence to the cortex. A large proportion of the sensory cortex is taken up by sensation from the face, especially the mouth and tongue, and from the hand, especially the thumb and first finger. This may in part be responsible for the common complaints of abnormalities of head and neck sensation, especially head and neck pain.

The integrity of the parietal lobes is always responsible for normal perception of the body image. If there is loss of parietal function, extinction may occur. The patient will deny appreciation of sensation of the body subserved by the diseased parietal lobe when bilateral sensory testing is performed.

REFLEXES

It is important to remember the concepts of upper motor neuron and lower motor neuron disease. The upper motor neuron system organizes groups of muscles to mediate movement of body parts. The lower motor neuron system organizes individual muscles.

Deep Tendon Reflexes and Superficial Reflexes

- Achilles reflex: S-1,2
- Quadriceps reflex: L-2,3,4
- Low abdominal: T-11, L-1
- Upper abdominal: T-6, T-9
- Hoffman reflex: C-7, C-8, and T1
- Brachioradialis reflex: C-5,6
- Biceps reflex: C-5, C-6
- Triceps reflex: C-6,7,8
- Jaw reflex: midpons

Those numbered segments underlined indicate the dominant or main spinal segments involved.

If present, pathologic reflexes are a sign of organic brain or spinal cord disease.

By testing the deep tendon reflexes as well as the superficial reflexes, one can sample the influences of both the upper motor neuron and the lower motor neuron on the reflex arcs. Beginning from the lower extremities and proceeding proximally, the plantar response depends on the intactness of the L-5 and S-1,2 segments. If the plantar response is extensor it indicates that the corticospinal pathway serving the L-5, S-1,2 segments has been disturbed.

CONCLUSION

In conclusion, an adequate history, a thorough physical examination and a competent neurologic examination usually enable the physician to make a correct headache diagnosis and do much toward reassuring the patient.

Reference

Graham JR (1974) Cluster headache. *Postgrad Med* 56: 181–185.

4

Additional Studies Are Sometimes Necessary in Investigating Headache

Many headache patients have had extensive diagnostic studies, particularly if their complaints are persistent and chronic, if they have responded poorly to prescribed therapy and if they have visited in many consultation rooms. Often such procedures have been done for what seem to be weak indications. But it is unwise to be too critical of others, for even when the attending physician has the best of intentions, patients with headache may be overtested, especially if the historic data hint at some form of obscure disease as a basis for their complaints. It is unfortunately true that some diagnostic studies, particularly arteriograms and pneumoencephalograms, may increase the patient's headache and more permanently fix in his mind the concern that serious organic disease of the brain is present.

Some diagnostic studies may increase the patient's headache.

Yet, on occasion, headache can be the first symptom of organic disease. If the patient is being seen for the first time for this complaint, some workup is indicated, unless history is crystal clear. We advise that skull films and, if the symptoms warrant it, computerized axial tomography (CT) and an electroencephalogram be performed on all patients with headache. This constitutes a baseline workup and is usually adequate to rule out organic disease. We proceed to more invasive studies including arteriography only if a specific indication for these procedures is present (Table 4.1). Chronic complaints of pain are *not* a specific indication.

It is important to disturb the patient as little as possible by your examinations and to reassure him by informing him when the tests are negative. If further investigations are indicated, make your patient understand the reasons for these studies and the risks involved, and obtain his consent for them.

SOME DIAGNOSTIC POINTS OF IMPORTANCE

Plain Skull Films

This procedure, although sometimes castigated as overused or unnecessary, does provide a large amount of clinical evidence, both positive and negative, of obvious and significant importance to the clinician caring for the patient with headache (Peterson, 1973). It is first necessary to make certain that the alignment of the films has been satisfactory. For example, on the lateral view the orbital plates and the mandibular rami should be superimposed, and on the anterior-posterior view the distances from the orbital rim to the outer bony table should be the same. The outer and inner table of the skull should be examined, as well as the lines and sutures, character and

Table 4.1. A View of the Headache "Workup"

General
- History and physical examination
- Skull films
- EEG

If focal disease, mass lesions or hydrocephalus is suspected
- CT scan and/or
- Brain scan

If arterial disease is suspected
- Angiograms

If infection is suspected
- Lumbar puncture, immediately

If temporal arteritis is suspected
- Sedimentation rate
- Temporal artery biopsy, antinuclear antibody (ANA)

Also, occasionally indicated in special situations
- X-rays of the temporomandibular joints—for chronic facial pain

If disease of cervical spine is suspected

Cervical spine films	
EMG	for signs of radiculopathy or spinal cord compression
Myelography, rarely	

density of the bones, the shape and size of the sella turcica, unusual calcifications (especially the pineal calcification) (Fig. 4.1), the soft tissues of the skull, and the craniocephalic index and the general vault-to-base relationships. The basal angle should be calculated, and signs of basilar impression should be sought.

The clinician should learn to identify, among other abnormalities,

- fractures
- splitting of the sutures
- increased digital markings suggesting increased intracranial pressure
- normal and pathologic vascular markings
- shifts of the calcified pineal gland
- other intracranial calcifications
- the abnormal range of sellar size (maximal internal AP diameter is 17 to 18 mm, average AP diameter is 10 mm)
- erosion of the sella
- metastatic disease (see Figure 2.3)

Some findings, such as subgaleal hematomas, can be recognized on skull films as benign and will usually disappear slowly without intervention.

Spinal Puncture

This should be done only if there is a specific indication. If the patient's neck is rigid and he is running a febrile course, a spinal puncture is mandatory to rule out intracranial infection. An increase of spinal fluid pressure is often present with a brain tumor and the spinal fluid pressure should be taken before any spinal fluid is withdrawn. Herniation of the brainstem into the foramen magnum and sudden death can occur if fluid is rapidly removed, if a brain tumor is present with associated increase in intracranial pressure. In general, if a brain tumor is seriously suspected as a cause of headache, spinal puncture is best avoided.

Electroencephalogram, Echoencephalogram

In some instances, an electroencephalogram may reveal a specific focal lesion, or dysrhythmia, suggestive that further studies should be done. If you are suspicious of a focal lesion or of organic disease of the brain, a negative electroencephalogram may be misleading. Echoencephalograms are used to assess the state of the midline structures. Lesions such as a unilateral subdural hematoma may shift the midline to the side opposite the lesion. If, however, bilateral lesions are present, the midline structures may not be shifted and this factor should be appreciated, particularly if there is a history of head trauma.

Computerized Axial Tomography (The CT Scan)

Most authorities agree that the CT scan, also termed the EMI scan, is the greatest advance in diagnostic medicine in the past several decades. This noninvasive technique uses a computer coupled with a special x-ray device to the produce vividly detailed cross-sectional pictures of the body's interior. The technique discloses variations in tissue density which aid in detecting many pathologic conditions.

The technique gives information about the brain and its appendages which previously could not be obtained or was obtained only with the greatest difficulty, using techniques such as pneumoencephalography, cerebral angiography, ventriculography or radioisotope scanning. In many cases, hazardous procedures such as pneumoencephalography and cerebral arteriography can now be avoided.

The CT scan makes it possible to differentiate hemorrhage from tumor, to follow multiple brain lesions, and to monitor chemotherapy, and the accuracy in diagnosing su-

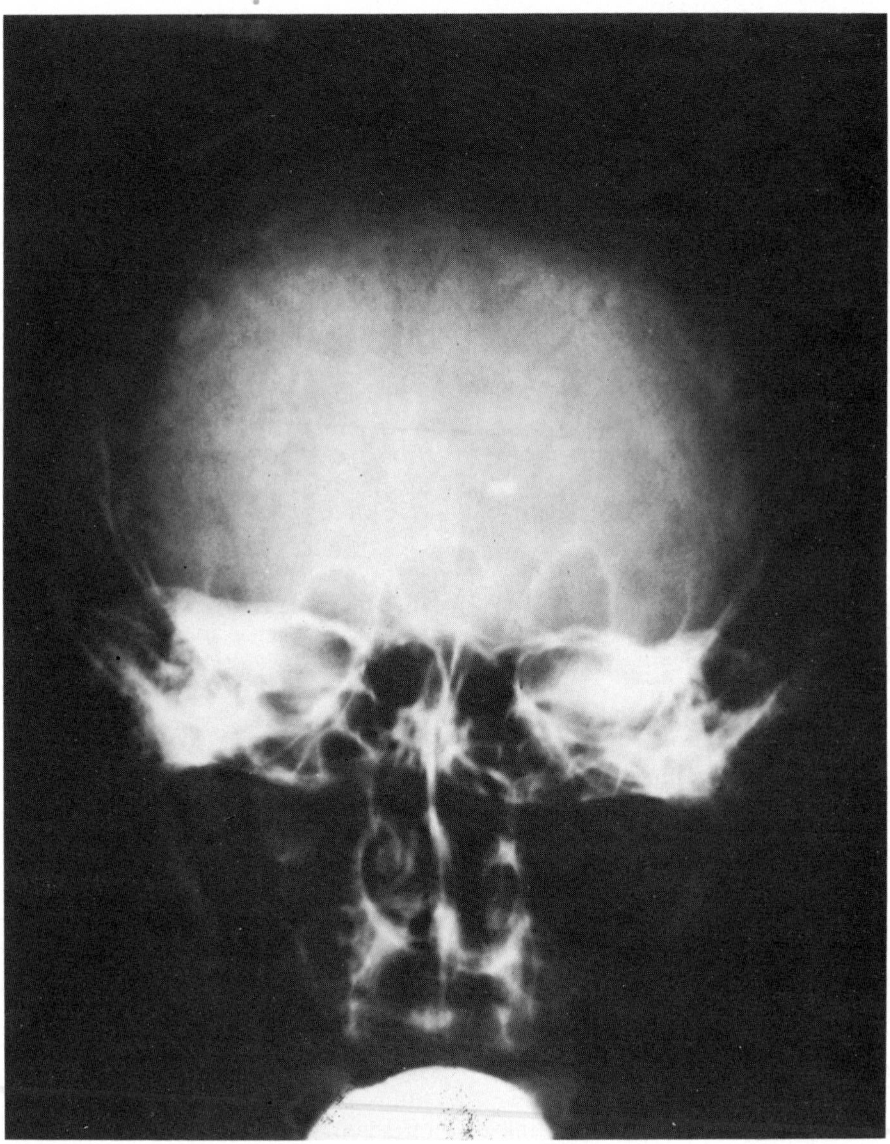

Figure 4.1. Routine skull films may reveal shift of the pineal gland. In this case the pineal gland is significantly shifted to the left, suggesting a mass in some part of the right hemisphere or atrophy on the left. Further neurologic diagnostic studies would be indicated.

pratentorial lesions surpasses that of previous techniques (Naidich, 1979). Furthermore, the testing can almost always be done on an outpatient basis, is rapid, does not overexpose the patient to irradiation, and is cost-effective (Evens et al., 1977).

In evaluation of the patient with headache, the CT scan is of particular value. It allows us to exclude conditions (including brain tumors, chronic subdural hematomas and hydrocephalus) which result in chronic recurrent headaches which at times simulate migraine. Also, for the first time, the CT scan has enabled us to recognize transient morphologic changes such as cerebral edema in the cerebral parenchyma after an acute attack of migraine, especially in cases of complicated migraine of the hemiparetic variety.

In a small percentage of patients with complicated migraine, abnormalities (including cerebral edema which is transient, lasting only a few days) will appear in CT scans; in addition, in patients with repeated severe attacks, cerebral ventricle enlargement and cerebral cortical atrophy have been reported (Hungerford, 1976).

The indications for the use of the CT scan in patients with recurrent headache are as follows:

- neurological examination suspicious for intracranial lesion
- recent onset of persistent headache, exertional headache, seizures or syncope, personality change
- change in character of headache.

See Figures 4-2 through 4-7.

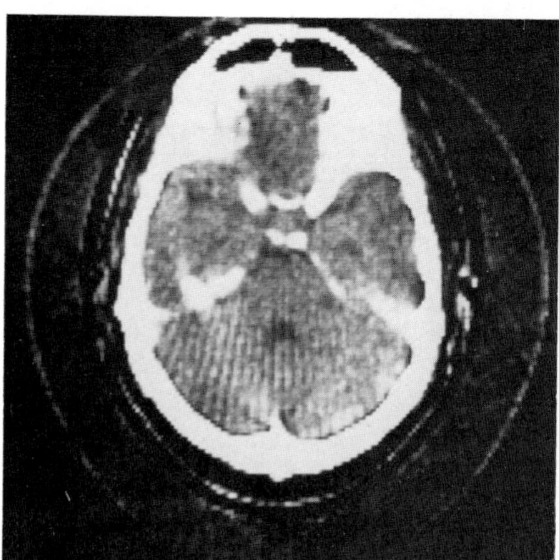
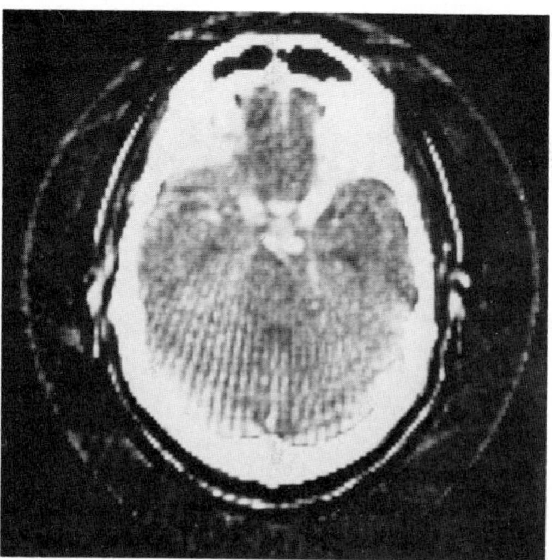

Figure 4.2. CT scan of a 70-year-old man with a history of recurrent vertex headaches, of moderate severity, often relieved by common analgesics. More troublesome was a history of recurrent episodes of severe sweating which were termed "male menopause." The CT scan demonstrates a pituitary tumor with contrast enhancement. The patient has been treated with radiation. A specific tissue diagnosis has not been obtained.

Radioactive Isotope Brain Scanning

The radioactive isotopes of mercury, technetium, and arsenic can be used for the visualization of lesions of the brain, including tumors, subdural hematomas, inflammatory masses, and vascular lesions. It may be especially useful as a second examination when the CT scan has proved negative and there is continued strong clinical suspicion of a lesion. Radioactive isotope scanning is a simple and noninvasive procedure, although limited by its relative expense. In general, it may be stated that the more vascular the lesion, the more consistent its demonstration will be using radioisotope techniques. Nonetheless, given the increasing value of CT scanning, particularly as new refinements appear, the

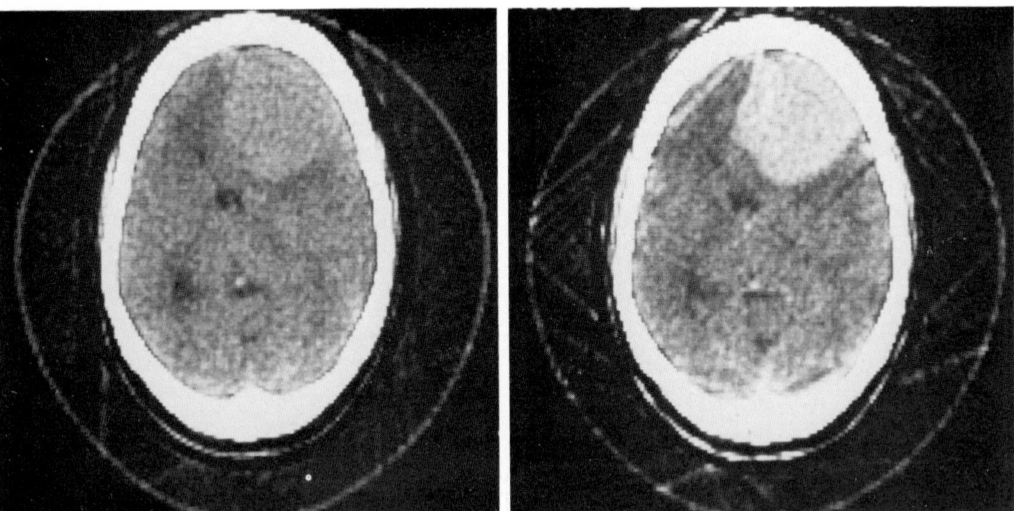

Figure 4.3. CT scan of an 18-year-old girl with a strong family history of vascular headache and with increasingly severe headaches for the past 3 months. No alteration with position or activity. No papilledema was present. The CT scan demonstrates a large tumor with contrast enhancement in the right frontal area. Pathological diagnosis was meningioma.

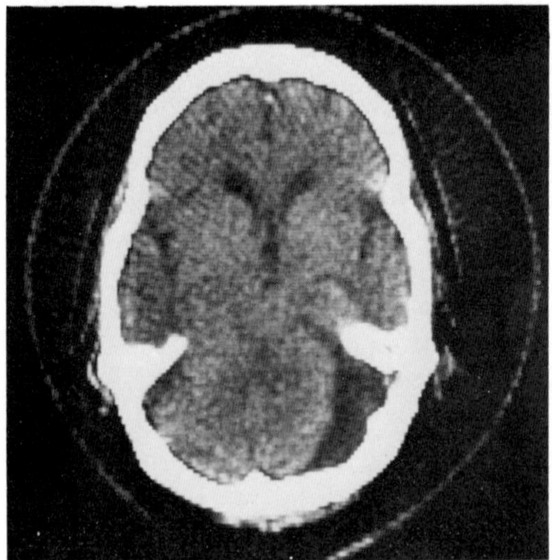

Figure 4.4. CT scan of an elderly man with a previous history of bilateral subdural hematomas, occurring 3 years prior to the onset of nonspecific occipital headaches, increasing somnolence and disorientation. The CT scan demonstrates a recurrent posterior subdural hematoma which was easily evacuated.

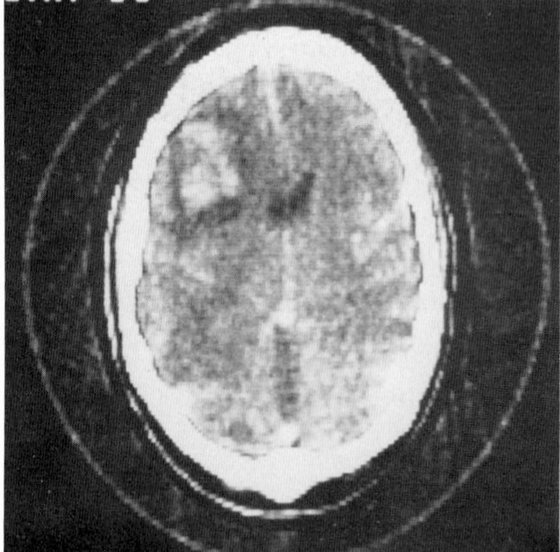

Figure 4.5. CT scan of a 27-year-old man with a strong family history of migraine referred because of increasing headaches, termed by his physician-father as migrainous. Note the large defect in the left frontal area with contrast enhancement. Pathological diagnosis was an astrocytoma Grade III.

use of radioisotope brain scanning in headache patients has declined.

Angiography

This is performed by a neuroradiologist, a neurosurgeon or a vascular surgeon and depicts aneurysms, angiomas, hematomas and pathologic circulation in tumors. It can be highly effective in localizing tumors, but the procedure is not without risk and should be used only when there is definite suspicion of an organic lesion. Angiography should be avoided, if possible, during episodes of migraine.

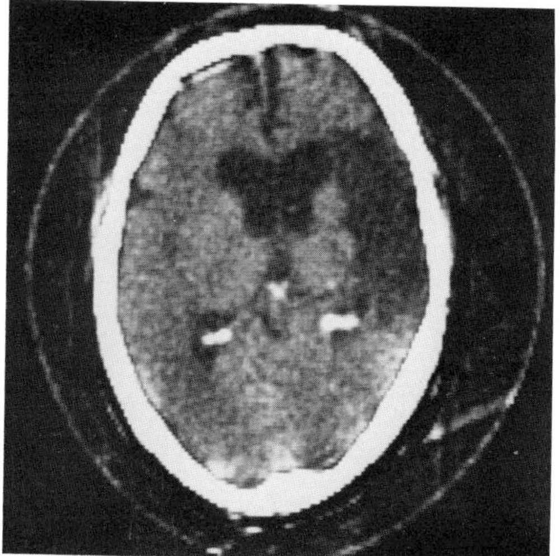

Figure 4.6. CT scan of a 54-year-old man complaining of nonspecific frontal and occipital headaches, with a previous history of a cerebrovascular accident and a persistent left hemiparesis. The CT scan shows a large lucent area in the right hemisphere compatible with the previous cerebral infarction.

Digital Subtraction Angiography (DSA)

In patients with transient ischemic attacks or carotid bruits, migraine-like headaches can be a symptom. Carotid angiography may increase the risk of stroke. A new noninvasive technique in which a computer translates pictures into numbers, DSA subtracts a preinjection image, called the mask, from later shots—as many as 30 every second—of the medium flowing through the artery. What is left, displayed instantly on the TV monitor, is an angiogram whose spatial resolution approaches that of catheter arteriography. Al-

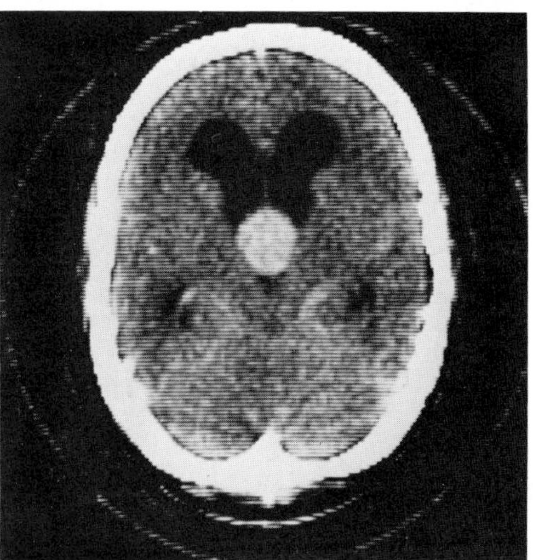

Figure 4.7. CT scan of J. W., a 36-year-old male, who noted the onset of severe headaches in November of 1974, with associated fatigue, lack of energy and weight loss in early 1975. In the past he had taken "handfulls" of aspirin for minor headaches but recently the headaches had become more severe and occurred several times per week, radiating from the occipital region to the frontal area. They were nonthrobbing but were associated with a sensation of pressure. Neurological examingation was normal. The discs were sharp. He appeared depressed. The initial CT scan shows massive dilation of the lateral ventricles, with the fourth ventricle of normal size. There is a mass density present in the region of the foramen of Monro. At operation this proved to be a colloid cyst of the third ventricle. His postoperative course was complicated by persistent hydrocephalus, and a ventriculo-peritoneal shunt was placed, subsequent to which he improved. He has remained relatively asymptomatic to the present time.

though the contrast-medium dose—and therefore the risk of reactions to it—is about the same as for standard angiography, there have been no deaths or strokes among the several thousand DSA patients so far. As this technique is improved, visualization of aneurysms may also be possible.

THE FUTURE OF IMAGING

CT scanning, so far used primarily as a superior x-ray device capable of displaying the human body in cross-sectional anatomy, can through dynamic spatial reconstruction be adapted to project three-dimensional computerized images of internal organs. This has already been accomplished, for example, with the heart. Using such techniques, it should be possible in the near future to visualize coronary arteries through intravenous contrast administration. Within the next decade, clinicians can look forward to three-dimensional pictures of the brain as a part of their diagnostic studies.

Positron Emission Transaxial Tomograph (PETT)

Large computer controlled tomographic units will also be able to map the distribution of positron-emitting radioisotopes and, thus, map out the function and physiology of organs. Such units are already in place and their use, while currently experimental, promises to further widen the horizons of clinicians. This instrument, termed the "positron emission transaxial tomograph" (PETT), requires large production facilities, including a cyclotron, in order to produce the required positron labeled chemicals (Ter-Pogossian, 1980).

Those chemicals currently in use include ammonia labeled with nitrogen-13, red blood cells labeled with carbon monoxide-11, ethylenediaminetetraacetic acid (EDTA) labeled with gallium, and carbon-11 palmitate. Such compounds have been used to survey brain, heart, and lung functions in experimental animals and in humans. Using the appropriate compound, for example, one can watch the visual cortex light up in response to light. Furthermore, metabolic abnormalities, without associated structural abnormalities, can sometimes be seen using PETT techniques. This is especially the case in brain function. In seizures, for example, an area of the brain can be shown to be hypometabolic during an interictal period and hypermetabolic at the time of the ictus (seizures) (Phelps, 1977; Ter-Pogossian, 1981).

Nuclear Magnetic Resonance (NMR)

A different form of investigative machine makes use of a strong magnetic field and radiofrequency scanning probes to obtain information regarding organs without subjecting them to radiation. This technique, termed "nuclear magnetic resonance" (NMR) spectroscopy, is already used in chemistry and atomic physics. It is based on the knowledge that the nucleus of an atom spins and that some nuclei carry a magnetic field. When such atoms are placed into the field of a strong magnet and radiated with a pulse of radio waves, the nuclei will respond with a signal of their own. Happily, in the nucleus of water, hydrogen behaves as the proton and gives the strongest reply when subjected to an exciting pulse, using NMR techniques. (Remember that water makes up the bulk of the human body). With technology already in use, the tissue is subjected to a strong, externally applied magnetic field, which forces the atomic nuclei with magnetic charges to align themselves. A burst of radioenergy is then applied at right angles to the magnetic field, forcing the nuclei out of alignment. Using a computer to focus and scan the radio waves, images are produced. This technique, also called "zeugmatography," is similar to the CT scan and images the body in cross-sectional anatomy (Lauterbur, 1973; Moore et al., 1980). But remember, again, that this is done without using x-ray and without the hazards of radiation.

Who will get these machines? Who will be able to afford them? PETT will be available only to a few institutions, given the huge organizational apparatus required to support it. NMR will probably be equivalent to CT in cost, and when perfected, NMR units can be expected to proliferate.

With machines such as these, the ability of physicians to work up patients in the year 2000, for example, is best left to our imaginations. None of us can even begin to anticipate what medicine will be like at that time, but surely diagnostic wonders await us.

ache from lactose ingestion as from the "offending" substance.

Diet for the Headache Patient
Avoid:
Ripened cheeses (cheddar, Emmentaler, Gruyere, Stilton, Brie and Camembert)
(Cheeses permissible: American, cottage, cream and Velveeta)
Herring
Chocolate
Vinegar (except white vinegar)
Anything fermented, pickled or marinated
Sour cream, yogurt
Nuts, peanut butter
Hot fresh breads, raised coffeecakes and doughnuts
Pods of broad beans (lima, navy and pea pods)
Any foods containing large amounts of monosodium glutamate (Chinese foods)
Onions
Canned figs
Citrus foods (no more than 1 orange per day)
Bananas (no more than ½ banana per day)
Pizza
Pork (no more than 2 or 3 times per week)
Excessive tea, coffee, cola beverages (no more than 4 cups per day)
Avocado
Fermented sausage (bologna, salami, pepperoni, summer and hot dogs)
Chicken livers
Avoid all alcoholic beverages, if possible. If you must drink, no more than two normal size drinks.
Suggested drinks: Haute Sauterne
Riesling
Seagram's VO
Cutty Sark
Vodka

Hypoglycemia

A word should be said about the quality and amount of food consumed by the patient with migraine. Hypoglycemia exerts a profound effect on the tone of the cranial blood vessels. If the sugar content of the blood is reduced by insulin or by other means, conspicuous cerebral vasodilation occurs. Headache is a prominent symptom of insulin shock, for example. Furthermore, in migraine patients, the relative hypoglycemia produced by fasting may evoke typical vascular headaches. Even reactive hypoglycemia occurring after ingestion of an excessive carbohydrate load may precipitate vascular headache in a susceptible person. For these reasons, we suggest that the patient with migraine eat three well-balanced meals a day and avoid an overabundance of carbohydrates at any single meal. Avoidance of oversleeping on weekends is also recommended. Excessive sleep may alter the body's normal blood sugar level and thus precipitate headaches when a rigid schedule of awakening is not kept.

HORMONAL CHANGES

Approximately 70% of the women seen with migraine say that some of their attacks occur prior to, during, or at the end of their menstruation. By the third month of pregnancy, most women are free of their migraine—except for a very small number who get their first attack with pregnancy.

The oral contraceptives and postmenopausal hormonal therapies usually increase the severity and frequency of migraine attacks (Dalton, 1975). Migraine patients appear to have an extremely labile vascular system and are subject to complications such as stroke from the use of oral contraceptives (Gardner et al., 1967).

ALLERGY, EPILEPSY AND MIGRAINE

We do not believe that there is any relationship between migraine and allergy or epilepsy. Migraine patients may note an increase in headache during or following an allergic episode, related to increased vasomotor activity. Presumably, also, the vasoconstrictive phase of migraine can set off seizure activity in one predisposed to seizures, but this series of events must be rare. EEG changes have been reported in migraine patients but their importance is conjectural. An occasional migraine patient with a significant dysrhythmia may respond to anticonvulsant agents.

Medina and Diamond (1976) have presented their studies on migraine and atopy. They determined serum IgE levels in 116 patients with headache by the radioimmunoassay technique. A second group consisted of 504 patients who were seen at a headache clinic during a period of 2 months. Elevation of the serum IgE was noted in 5.7% of the migraine population, approximately the same as the incidence of elevated serum IgE in the normal population. This incidence is far below that seen in atopic disorders. In the second group of 504 patients, the prevalence of atopic disorders in migraine patients and their relatives was approximately the same as the prevalence in patients with chronic muscle contraction headaches. The numbers are close to the prevalence of atopy in the normal population or their relatives and are not statistically significant. There is, therefore, no increase in the prevalence of atopy in the relatives of patients suffering from migraine headaches. This study casts further doubt on any supposed relationship between atopy, allergy, elevation of the serum IgE and migraine. It now seems evident, from this and other careful studies, that migraine is not an allergic phenomenon and is not related to the atopic diseases.

SITE AND CHARACTER OF HEADACHE

The most frequent history obtained is that of a dull ache, progressively worsening and finally developing into a throbbing or pulsating pain. As it becomes stabilized the headache may again become constant and nonthrobbing. About 70% of migraine is unilateral and frequently affects the frontal and temporal regions but may settle behind the eye. The pain can radiate across the head and to other regions of the face and neck surrounding the primary pain site.

NUMBER, DURATION AND ONSET OF ATTACKS

The number of attacks varies—in severe cases, attacks may occur every few days; in moderate cases, attacks may occur only once or twice a year. Most frequently, patients report two to four attacks monthly. Most migraine episodes last longer than 4 hours, usually for a day or two. A severe attack can last up to 6 days. The onset can occur at any time and may be precipitated by various factors. It is not uncommon for a migraine patient to wake up with a headache.

THE ATTACK

In the initial phase of migraine, during the prodromal phase, there is vasoconstriction, followed by vasodilation, during which the headache occurs. In about 35% of cases, the patient has the typical classic migraine described above. The patient notes an aura (most often visual) which may precede the attack by 10–20 minutes. Then the typical one-sided, pulsating headache occurs with its associated symptoms. Nonclassic migraine does not have preheadache prodromes.

PRODROMES IN ORDER OF FREQUENCY

The prodromes in order of frequency are

1. Scotomata, or blind spots
2. Teichopsia, or fortification spectra—a zigzag pattern resembling a fort (Fig. 5.3)
3. Flashing of lights (photopsia) light-colored
4. Paresthesias
5. Visual and auditory hallucinations; Alice in Wonderland syndrome described by Lewis Carroll, a sufferer from migraine, who saw the distorted figures of "Alice" as part of his migraine attack (Fig. 5.4).

OTHER RARE PRODROMES

Diplopia, ataxia, vertigo, syncope and hyperosmia may occur. The prodromes usually resolve before each attack but can, on occasion, remain permanent. As a migraine sufferer grows older he may note only the prodrome without the subsequent headache.

SYMPTOMS ACCOMPANYING MIGRAINE ATTACKS

- Photophobia—Undue sensitivity to light, preferring darkened room. Noise can also increase discomfort.

In polyarteritis nodosa, there are multiple areas of arterial necrosis and inflammation affecting many organs. The arterial lesion appears to be identical to that found in serum sickness. γ-Globulin may be identified in areas of fibrinoid necrosis. The role of this γ-globulin in the production of the arterial lesion is the subject of intensive investigation. Some patients with biopsy-proven polyarteritis have Australia antigenemia, suggesting that an immunologic reaction to a virus or virus-like particle had produced the systemic vasculitis. Circulating immune complexes are found in these patients and are composed of Australia antigen and immunoglobulin. Studies of tissue from 1 patient showed deposition of Australia antigen, IgM and β1C in blood vessel walls.

In temporal arteritis, a similar pathologic picture occurs, except that the inflammatory reaction may be limited to the cranial arteries. The elastic tissues appear frayed or fragmented, and giant cells within the vessel walls are almost a constant feature of the pathologic findings. The giant cells are most numerous in the region of the deranged internal elastic lamina.

We have surveyed 36 temporal artery biopsies obtained during the calendar years 1975 through 1978. All were examined with standard pathological techniques, with hematoxylin and eosin (H&E) and with immunofluorescence (IF). Of the 36 patients, 21 were female and 15 were male. The paraffin sections were evaluated by H&E and, in some selected cases, elastic stains. IF included IgG, IgA, IgM, Cl_q, C3 and fibrinogen. Nine patients had evidence of immunologic reactivity and/or components in their temporal arteries.

In addition, there were 8 additional cases with H&E or IF only. Of these 8 additional cases, 4 showed fibrinogen within the lumen and IgG on the internal elastic membrane.

Not all patients with "temporal arteritis" have headache, but when present the headache is of high intensity, of a deep aching quality, throbbing in nature, and persistent (Fig. 8.3; Plate 14.7). In addition to the aching and throbbing, there is often a burning component, unlike most other vascular headaches. The headache is slightly worse when the patient lies flat in bed and is diminished in intensity by the upright or half upright position. It is somewhat reduced in intensity by digital pressure on the common carotid artery on the affected side and is made worse by stooping over. There is hyperalgesia of the scalp and the distended arteries are extremely tender, so that any pressure greatly increases the pain.

Some patients may suffer pain on mastication, and in some it may be the initial symptom. Facial swelling and redness of the skin overlying the temporal arteries, with the addition of the burning component of pain, are usually noted after the onset of headache. Immediate relief from burning pain and headache may follow biopsy of the inflamed temporal artery, and it is assumed that this follows the interruption of the afferents for pain about the vessel.

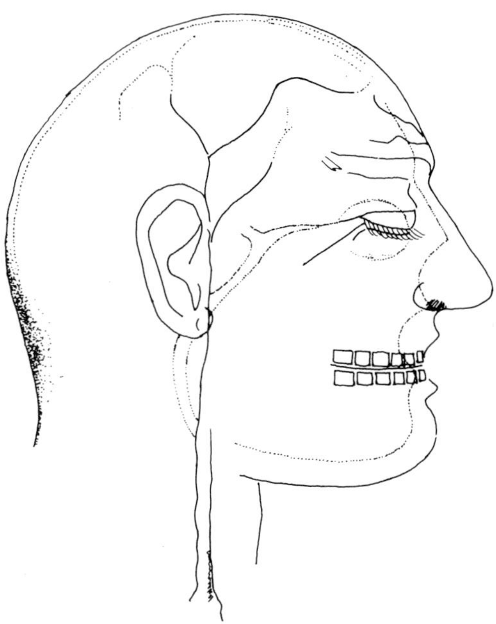

Figure 8.3. Clinical features of cranial (temporal) arteritis: often unilateral headache; temporal artery is sometimes enlarged, rigid and tender; sudden or gradual loss of vision in one eye if the ophthalmic artery is involved. Early possible complaints include pain in the ear, pain with chewing, pain in the teeth and sometimes pain in the occiput.

Prior to the onset of the full-blown picture

of "temporal arteritis," there often is pain in the teeth, ear, jaw, zygoma and nuchal region and occiput. The distribution of these symptoms suggests primary involvement of other branches of the external carotid artery, notably the external and internal maxillary arteries.

Other arteries may also be involved, including the major vessels of the aorta, the coronaries, and the arteries of the limbs. Large- and medium-sized arteries are the principal sites of the inflammatory process. Aneurysm formation may occur in association with the arteritis.

The presenting complaint may be of ocular symptoms. It has become evident that more than a third of patients with temporal arteritis are threatened with partial or even complete loss of vision. Diplopia and photophobia have been noted, and ophthalmoscopic evidence of occlusion of the ophthalmic artery has been apparent in some cases.

Some patients have presented signs suggestive of cerebral damage and encephalitis during the acute stage of the illness. We have observed several patients with thrombotic strokes related to cranial arteries. Other atypical presentations of temporal arteritis have been reported by Paulley and Hughes (1960).

If loss of vision is the presenting complaint, then a medical emergency is in progress and the patient requires urgent treatment. This should not wait upon the specific method used to make the diagnosis, that of temporal artery biopsy. Prednisone or some other corticosteroid is the treatment of choice. As soon as the diagnosis is made, 40 to 60 mg should be given. The sedimentation rate should be followed as a guide to management with prednisone. It is generally necessary to continue therapy with prednisone at a low maintenance dose of approximately 10–20 mg for a prolonged period.

PAINFUL OPHTHALMOPLEGIA (TOLOSA-HUNT SYNDROME)

Painful ophthalmoplegia, as the name implies, is a rare syndrome characterized by eye muscle paresis and pain. It is a chronic inflammatory process of unknown etiology, which usually involves the cavernous sinus, the carotid artery, the orbit, and, at times, the clivus and the middle cranial fossa. Often it begins with pain, followed by ophthalmoplegia and marked elevation of the erythrocyte sedimentation rate. The sympathetic nervous system may be involved, producing a Horner's syndrome. The optic nerve may be involved. The process may be self-limited or may recur. A good response to corticosteroids is the rule.

Other conditions which produce painful ophthalmoplegia need to be excluded. A computed tomography (CT) scan of the orbit is a particularly useful diagnostic study in this situation.

Occasional reports of cases of Tolosa-Hunt syndrome still appear in the medical literature. Smith and Taxdal (1966) have emphasized the dramatic response of the syndrome to systemic corticosteroid therapy. Recently Takeoka et al. (1978) have described angiographic findings in a patient with the Tolosa-Hunt syndrome. During the acute episode, at a time when a right third nerve paresis was present, there was evidence of irregular narrowing in the carotid siphon and incomplete opacification of the anterior cerebral artery. Ten days later, after treatment with corticosteroids, there was a remarkable improvement in the prior stenosis.

A few observations on the Tolosa-Hunt syndrome deserve emphasis. There is a close relationship between the oculomotor paresis which occurs and the angiographic abnormalities. In most patients, pupillary function remains normal, with only 20% showing some pupillary involvement. The onset of the third nerve paresis is rather rapid, but complete recovery almost always results when appropriate therapy is provided.

DISEASE OF THE CRANIAL OR NECK STRUCTURES

Headache may be related to diseases of the eyes, nose, teeth or any of the other structures of the head. Noxious stimuli can be elicited by localized pressure phenomena, muscle contraction, trauma, tumor or inflammation. Generally, these headaches are confined to the affected area, although occasionally, due to central spread of excitation, their effects may be appreciated in more distant regions of the skull. Persistent painful stimuli may lower pain threshold and so evoke other forms of headache. For example, pain from ocular disease can be related to several different mechanisms and thus present a diagnostic challenge to the clinician. Eye pain may occur with increased ocular pressure, traction on ocular muscles, inflammation of the eye tissues, hyperopia or astigmatism, exposure to light, new growths or trauma (Fig. 8.4). In pseudotumor of the orbit, there is severe pain together with ophthalmoplegia, usually the result of an inflammatory lesion of the cavernous sinus or of the orbit itself.

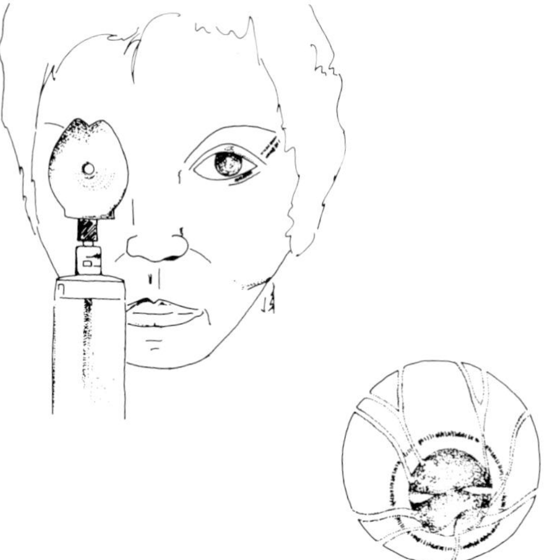

Figure 8.4. Clinical features of glaucoma: intense headache involving the eye and supraorbital area; glaucomatous cupping of the optic disc; dilated pupil; pain in the eyeball; increased intraocular pressure.

Headache related to nasal disease is usually anterior and is often related to nasal vasomotor phenomena. The symptoms include local pain and discomfort. Demonstration of a precise paranasal disease, such as sinusitis or allergic rhinitis, usually removes the headache from this category. This form of headache is frequently associated with vasomotor rhinitis and is assumed to represent a localized vascular reaction to stress.

HEADACHE AND THE EYE

Ocular pain may occur as an isolated area of pain or may be referred from contiguous structures. Most ocular pains are due to primary disorders of the eye or orbit and include glaucoma, anterior uveitis, corneal ulcer, and the like. Obviously, disorders such as these should be managed by the ophthalmologist. If there is any question regarding eye disease, because of eye pain, an ophthalmological consultation is mandatory.

Believing that they need new glasses, many patients with headache localized to the eyes or even with generalized headache will present first to an optometrist or ophthalmologist. There probably are symptoms associated with eye strain, particularly with refractive errors or ocular motor disturbances. Such headaches are accompanied by complaints of pain, fatigue, and discomfort, associated with sustained visual effort, and should prove to be no problem to the alert clinician. Again, ophthalmologic referral is indicated.

Many ocular pains are referred or represent pain of another specific process. Perhaps the most frequent causes of referred eye pain and visual disturbances are vascular headaches, either migraine or cluster headache. Ocular pain may also occur with isolated ocular muscle palsy, with cranial arteritis, with cavernous sinus lesions of varying types, and in orbital ischemia (Lyle, 1968).

HEADACHE AND SINUSITIS

Many patients with chronic headaches insist that the headaches are related to sinusitis or are, in fact, sinus headaches. This is invariably incorrect. Chronic recurring headache in an otherwise asymptomatic patient rarely arises in the ear, nose, or throat areas. Inflammation of the paranasal sinuses, ears, or pharynx will cause localized and quite acute pain, but generally the pattern of the pain will parallel the course of the illness, which is often associated with systemic signs of disease, including fever, sweats, and, if prolonged, weight loss. Occasionally, an indolent disease of a sinus (such as a mucocele or an osteoma) or even a chronic fungus infection (such as actinomycosis) may produce chronic pain, but this is an unlikely occurrence.

Usually the patient reports to the otolaryngologist because either the patient, his family, or his physician believes that the headache may be due to organic disease particularly involving the ears, nose, throat or sinuses. The diagnostic workup endeavors to prove or disprove this concept. Paranasal sinus films are indicated, and multiple views need to be taken. Tomography may be necessary if one wishes to demonstrate a localized bony erosion of the walls of a sinus. CT scans can be used to delineate soft tissue masses in the sinuses and their relationships to the orbit, central nervous system and other adjacent structures.

Nasopharyngeal carcinoma may be an occult disease with subtle signs and may cause headache for a prolonged period before it is discovered. Nasopharyngeal carcinomas have an uneven growth pattern and may be seen in young adults or even children. Here again, an adequate physical examination of the nasopharynx by a skilled clinician using a mirror is mandatory. Direct examination and biopsy under general anesthesia is frequently required to secure a diagnosis. Tomography of the base of the skull may show areas of erosion.

In general, the diagnostic workup for nasal disease producing headache should be managed by a physician skilled in dealing with this area. An adequate physical examination with careful inspection of the nose is an absolute requirement. Patients with anterior head pain who are convinced that they have "sinus headaches" should have paranasal sinus films as well as a thorough physical examination. If there is any suspicion of more serious disease, then further workup is indicated. In general, however, it is unwise to correct minor abnormalities of nasal structures if the chief complaint is headache and no specific disease can be found.

CRANIAL NEURITIS AND NEURALGIAS AND TEMPOROMANDIBULAR JOINT (TMJ) DISEASE

Some forms of facial pain are considered to be related to the cranial nerves, excluding the trigeminal and glossopharyngeal neuralgias. They commonly include the atypical facial neuralgias, lower-half headache, vidian neuralgias, carotidynia and buccal neuralgia. Some of these syndromes are poorly developed and may not deserve a separate status. Some of them probably represent vascular pain or a form of migraine perceived in an unusual location. This is particularly true of lower-half headaches, which may respond to prophylaxis—as with lysergic acid derivatives such as methysergide.

Are there symptoms related to TMJ disease? The question is still being debated. We believe that facial pain can occur with TMJ disease, usually best appreciated locally, with radiation to the jaw, the neck and behind the ear, and not neuritic in character. In our view, the syndrome consists of localized facial pain, limitation of motion of the jaw, muscle tenderness and joint crepitus. Usually the joint itself is normal in its radiologic appearance.

The temporomandibular joint (TMJ) is the only moveable joint in the head, if one excludes the junction of the head with the atlas. The most common complaint in TMJ disease is headache, of moderate intensity and located at the vertex, occiput or in the face overlying the joints. Diagnosis may sometimes be difficult. One should certainly palpate and auscultate the joints with significant pressure, with the patient opening and closing his mouth. If crepitus can be heard, osteoarthritis in the joint can be assumed. One may thereafter inject a local anesthetic such as 1 cc of a 2% solution of lidocaine into the joint to see whether or not there is alteration in facial pain. Here again, consultation with a dentist who is knowledgeable in this field is essential. The point to be made is that patients with TMJ disease have pain primarily from muscular tension related to dental occlusive disease. Because of localized pain the patient begins to use the opposite side of the mouth on which to chew, attempting to splint the painful side but, in point of fact, this has exactly the opposite effect and makes the painful joint do all the work. For example, with right TMJ disease, chewing on the left side moves the right temporomandibular joint excessively. There is no evidence that hearing loss, damage to cranial nerves, disturbances of equilibrium, development of Ménière's syndrome or difficulty with the eustachian tubes is in any way related to this syndrome. Current concepts of etiology are that occlusal disharmony and psychophysiologic factors play primary roles, with most of the dysfunction resident in the masticatory

10

Headache in Children

Headache in children is a special subject and so deserves a special chapter. As with adults with headache, the large majority of children complaining of headache do not have organic disease as a basis for their complaints. Here again their headaches can be classified into three types: vascular, muscle contraction and traction and inflammatory (Table 10.1).

MIGRAINE

Vascular headaches in children may be classic in character, with premonitory symptoms, especially scotomata, followed by unilateral head pain. Severe nausea and hyperemesis are common in childhood migraine. Often the child appears pale, is obviously ill and "pasty," and usually retires to bed. Frequently also, the pain may be bilateral, rather than unilateral (Table 10.2).

In addition, however, some migrainous episodes may occur in childhood in a considerably more recondite manner. Ehyai and Fenichel (1978) have described 5 patients with acute confusional migraine in whom the primary complaint was one of confused agitation resembling a toxic metabolic psychosis. This syndrome occurred in both sexes between the ages of 5 and 16 years. An acute confusional state was the initial manifestation in one of their migrainous patients and in several children with this syndrome reported previously. In the absence of a history of migraine, there is considerable difficulty in making the diagnosis and thus a family history positive for migraine becomes an important clue. Headache may not be reported as a part of the acute confusional migraine syndrome, but typical migraine headaches always develop eventually. Confusion and disorientation are accompanied by agitation, a mixture of apprehension and combativeness. The duration of an attack is usually several hours but may be as brief as 10 minutes or as long as 20 hours. The episode usually terminates in a deep sleep and on awakening the children appear to be normal. Of their 5 patients, 4 had recurrent episodes of acute confusional migraine that tended to cluster over a relatively brief period of days or months. The mechanism is believed to be cerebral ischemia of one or both hemispheres. In general, no specific therapy is required for acute confusional migraine beyond reassurance of the family and patient of the benign nature of the attack and its relationship to the migraine process. Ergot compounds are not necessarily helpful since many of the complaints are thought to be related to intracranial vasoconstriction. Should vascular headache appear subsequent to the development of acute confusional migraine, ergot compounds in standard doses can be employed.

In a similar vein, Swanson and Vick (1978) reported 12 patients with basilar artery migraine and demonstrated an attack recorded electroencephalographically. They noted that basilar artery migraine was a distinctive disorder characterized by symptoms referable to dysfunction of brainstem structures in conjunction with more typical migrainous phenomena. In one patient, an attack of basilar artery migraine was captured during an electroencephalographic tracing and appeared as a typical photoconvulsive episode. The authors advised that greater than half their patients responded well to anticonvulsant drugs, particularly phenytoin. In basilar migraine there are a variety of brainstem, cerebellar and occipital cortical symptoms in association with the usual migrainous complaints. Loss of consciousness is common although not necessary for the diagnosis. When it occurs it is invariably brief and akinetic. There is some relationship between this syndrome and that described above of protracted confusional episodes; both are perhaps associated with vasomotor disturbances in the basilar artery.

Sillanpaa (1975) reported on the prevalence of headache in Finnish children starting school. In the two Finnish cities of Tampere and Turku, there were 4825 children, aged 7 years, who started their primary school in the autumn of 1974. At the first clinical examination performed by school doctors, 87.8% of the pupils and their mothers were interviewed to detect the occurrence of headache. The overall prevalence of headache proved to be 37.7%. Occasional headache, which was considered to be significant, was found in 32.7%. More frequent headache, occurring once a month or more, was found in 6.0% of cases. The prevalence of migraine was 3%. This contrasts with the study of Bille (1962) done in Upsala in 1962 on 9000 school children, in which 39% were found to have headaches. On the other hand, the present study showed a twofold higher frequency of migraine (3%) compared to Bille's series (1.4%).

It is important to realize that juvenile head trauma syndromes may be related to migraine and that migraine may occur after head trauma, particularly after trauma sustained in sporting activities such as football and baseball. Haas and his associates (1969, 1975) describe a clinical spectrum of juvenile head trauma in an analysis of 50 attacks in 25 patients. Attacks were grouped into four clinical types: 1) hemiparetic, 2) somnolent, 3) blindness and 4) brainstem signs. They suggest that these four types of juvenile head trauma syndromes are different manifestations of a common underlying process. All attacks followed mild head trauma after a latent interval, generally of 1 to 10 minutes. Forty of the 50 attacks occurred in patients

Table 10.1. Headache in Children

	Vascular (Migraine)	Muscle Contraction	Traction and Inflammatory (Increased Intracranial Pressure)
Sex	Males 2:1	Females 3:1	No sex differential
Age at onset	4–14 years	6–12 years	Any age
Prodromata	Scotomata, pallor, abdominal complaints, malaise, irritability	None	None
Associated findings	Nausea, vomiting, hyperemesis, confusional state	Avoids school or other stress situations	Vomiting, lethargy, positive neurologic signs, progressive head pain
Family history	Positive for migraine	Disturbed relationships	None

Table 10.2. Migraine in Children

Sex	Male:Female 2:1
Age at onset	4–14 years
Prodromata	Scotomata, pallor, abdominal complaints, malaise, irritability
Unusual manifestations	Confusion, agitation, apprehension, combativeness
Predisposing factors	Family history, head trauma
EEG	Often abnormal, may be dysrhythmic in basilar migraine

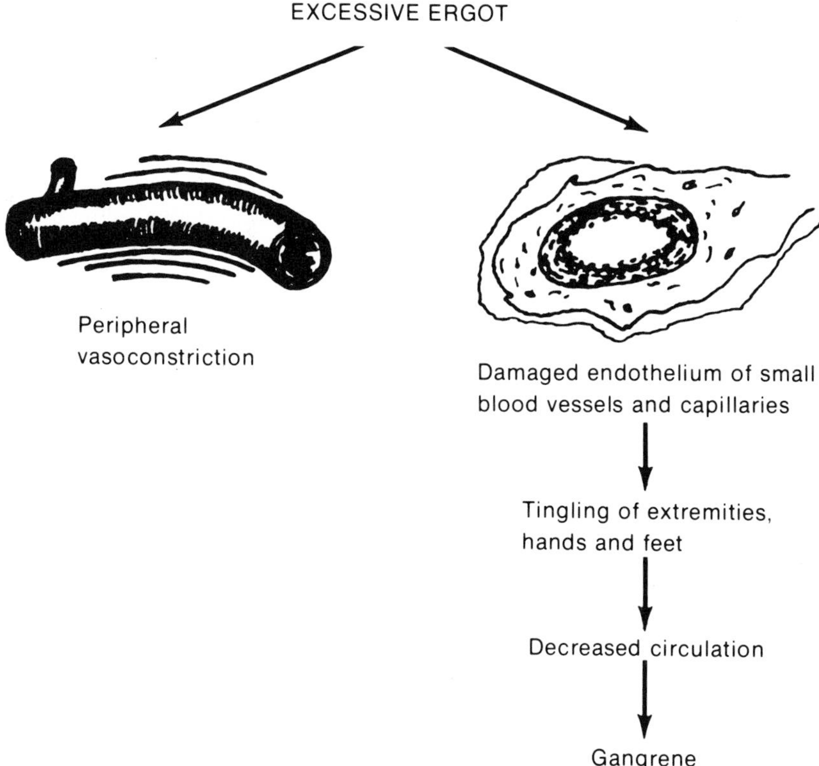

Figure 11.2. Ergotism. Any artery may be involved, including peripheral arteries, coronary arteries, and visceral arteries.

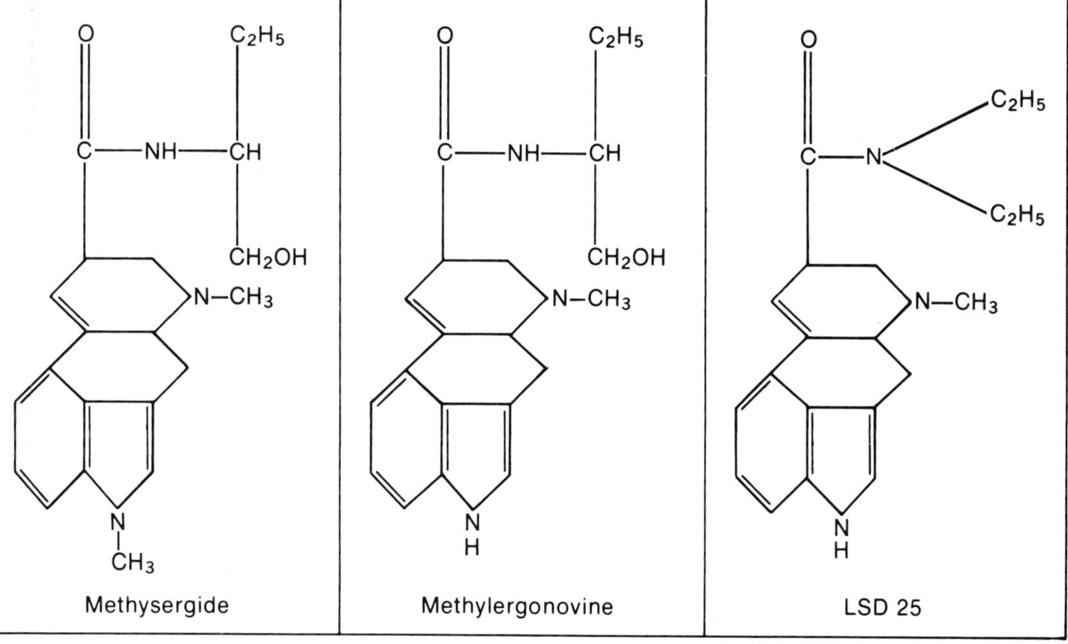

Figure 11.3. Common ergot compounds.

poisoning appeared. The disease occurred then in epidemics and was characterized primarily by symptoms of ischemia, including tingling, burning, numbness and claudication, followed by gangrene of the hands, feet and legs (Fig. 11.2). The illness had significant religious connotations. It was suggested that a type of Holy Fire was consuming the body. Subsequently, the name "St. Anthony's Fire" was also used, since a visitation to the Shrine of St. Anthony was sometimes curative. It is interesting that persons with ergotism were given a diet free of contaminated grain at the shrine and often recovered, further enhancing the belief in a divine cure. In addition to symptoms of peripheral ischemia, abortion was common with ergotism. Also, a form of ergotism associated with major motor seizures was described in those ancient epidemics of ischemia. In spite of this knowledge, outbreaks of ergot poisoning related to contamination of grain with the ergot fungus have continued.

The pharmacologic effects of the ergot compounds are complex, but for purposes of this discussion we will concentrate on their vascular effects. Ergotamine tartrate and related alkaloids produce peripheral vasoconstriction and also damage the endothelium of the capillaries and small blood vessels. Vascular stasis, thrombosis and gangrene may then ensue. The various ergot alkaloids differ significantly in these vasoconstrictor properties. Ergotamine is the most potent. Its effect in migraine is related largely to its vasoconstrictor properties.

Ergotamine tartrate is generally considered effective and safe in recommended doses but can damage blood vessels.

Ergotamine tartrate is generally considered to be safe when used in its recommended dose, and migraine patients tolerate ergot well. If more than 10–12 mg per week are taken by mouth, however, or more than 1 ml per day parenterally, side effects may occur. These are usually not dangerous and include nausea, vomiting, severe thirst and other gastrointestinal discomforts. In chronic ergot poisoning, however, very striking and significant circulatory changes may occur. The distal extremities become cold, pale and numb, with slight sweating of the feet. Claudication becomes evident. The patient may complain of unusual susceptibility to the cold. Arterial pulses eventually disappear and gangrene may ensue. Since ergot is a nonspecific vasoconstrictor and may affect other arteries, including the coronary arteries, angina pectoris may appear and electrocardiographic changes have been documented. The visceral arteries may also be affected.

Unusual sensitivity to ergot therapy may appear in:

- febrile states
- liver disease
- persons with compromised peripheral circulation

We therefore make it a rule never to employ ergot therapy in any patient with significant cardiovascular complaints and, in general, we avoid using the drug in persons over the age of 65 years.

Severe vasospasm may thus occur following ergot administration. Occasionally, this may be related to overdose. Patients particularly susceptible to ergot may develop profound vasoconstriction, as, for example, with Raynaud's disease.

Intravenous sodium nitroprusside may be helpful in patients in whom the signs and symptoms of peripheral ischemia are severe. The dose is 50 μg per minute, administered by a constant infusion pump, with careful monitoring of blood pressure in order to prevent hypotension. Chemical sympathectomy by lumbar and cervicothoracic sympathetic ganglion blockade may also be attempted in these patients and may prove to be therapeutic. Most often, watchful waiting, provision for symptomatic care, and withdrawal from ergot are the only treatment measures necessary.

METHYSERGIDE

Methysergide is, in fact, a methylated form of methylergonovine (Fig. 11.3). It is of value in headache prophylaxis by virtue of multiple sites of action (Fig. 11.4).

- When administered alone, methysergide may produce vasoconstriction.
- When administered with catecholamines and some other vasoconstrictor agents, methysergide acts synergistically to increase peripheral vasoconstriction.
- When administered either intravenously or by mouth, methysergide inhibits or alters the magnitude of central vasomotor reflexes.

Methysergide may also cause fibrosis of various areas of the body, which is relatively uncommon but is of sufficient intensity to cause great concern and to limit the usefulness of this drug in therapeutic situations (Graham, 1967). The most common fibrotic lesion produced has been retroperitoneal fibrosis, sometimes leading to the compromise of the the kidneys and to progressive renal failure. In addition, fibrosis has been observed in other areas, including the lungs and heart. The mechanism by which fibrosis is produced is unknown. Although methysergide is a powerful serotonin inhibitor, it has been suggested that it may, at times, act as a false serotonin transmitter (Fig. 11.5). In diseases characterized by serotonin excess, such as the carcinoid syndrome, fibrosis does occur, particularly in the myocardium, but retroperitoneal fibrosis in the carcinoid syndrome is unusual.

Given the tendency of methysergide to produce fibrosis, it should be used sparingly and with care by the physician. We usually recommend that it not be used for longer than 90 days. If it is used for a longer period, the drug should be stopped for a full month every 6 months, at which time a careful reevaluation of the patient is mandatory. Renal function studies and a chest x-ray should probably be done at these times.

OTHER DRUGS

Significant problems with analgesic abuse may appear with other medications and a thorough discussion of all of them is beyond the scope of this chapter. However, some general statements with respect to individual compounds can be made:

1. Compounds containing barbiturates have a significant capacity for addiction.

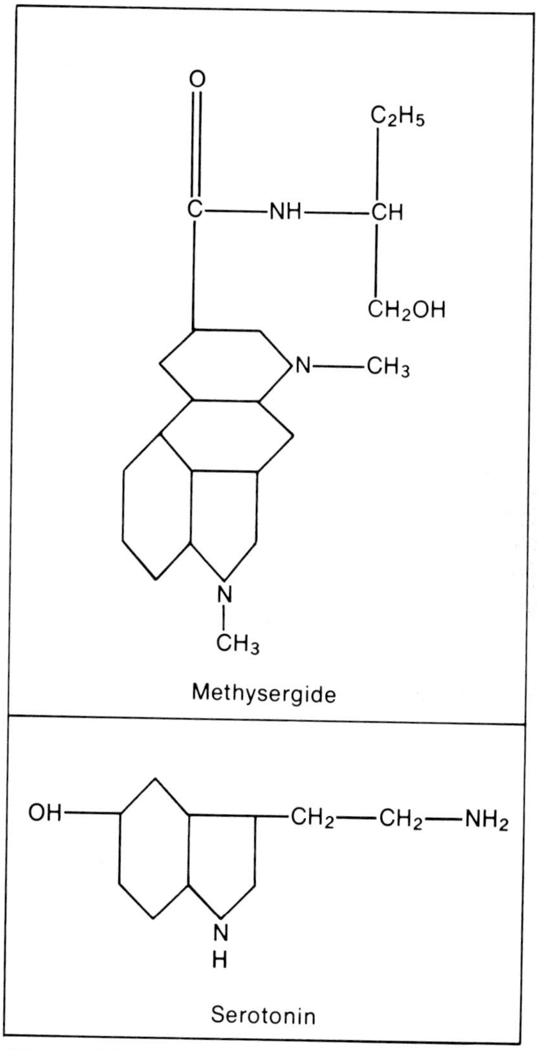

Figure 11.4. Structural formulas of methysergide and serotonin.

2. Monoamine oxidase (MAO) inhibitors may produce severe headache and hypertensive reactions if ingested with even small amounts of catecholamines.

Patients taking these medications need careful guidance regarding diet and other therapy. Aged cheese contains tyramine which if ingested while employing a MAO inhibitor may produce a severe hypertensive crisis. Even the small amounts of catecholamines

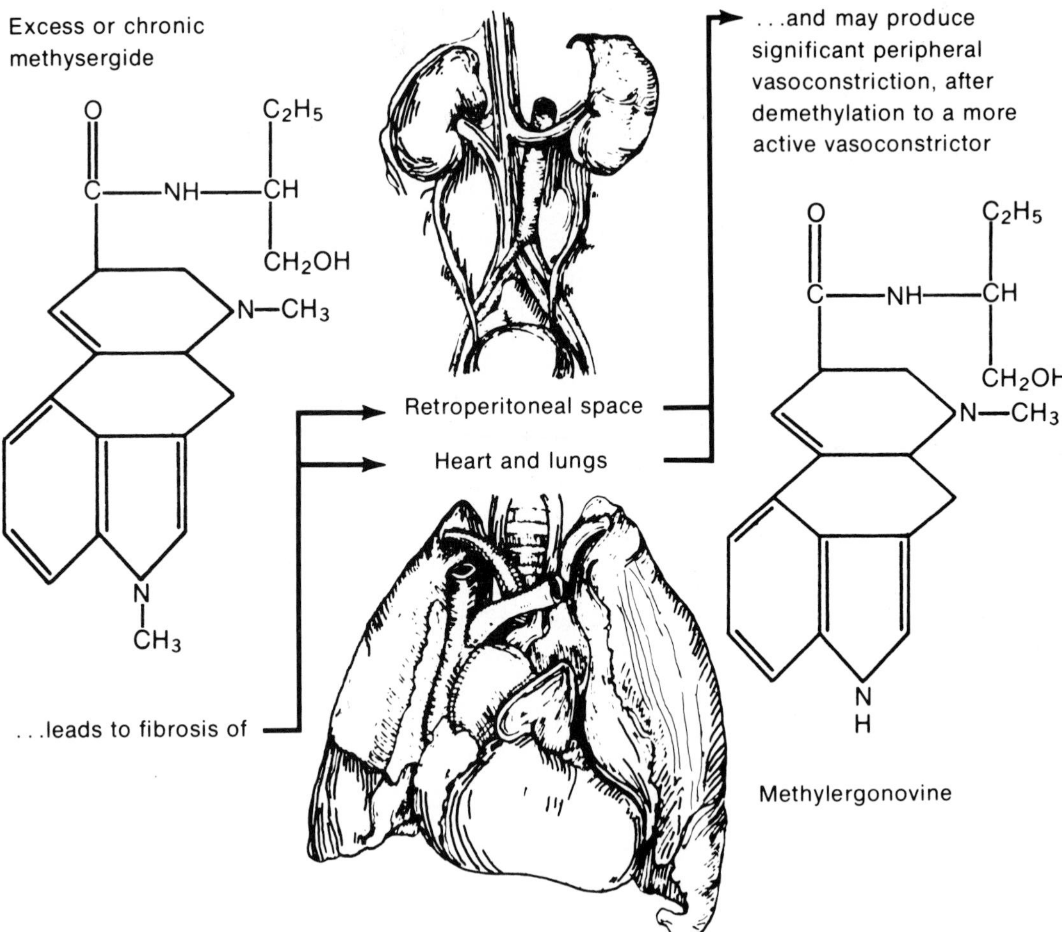

Figure 11.5. Methysergide toxicity.

present in proprietary cold pills and similar remedies should be avoided in this situation.

3. Phenothiazines are only occasionally abused in headache patients, but acute dystonic reactions may occur in some situations and must be recognized by the clinician. Tardive dyskinesia is an especially serious complication of long-term neuroleptic use.
4. Narcotics should not be given to patients with chronic headache. Addiction potential is especially significant in patients in whom the pain is chronic and not acute and in whom a tendency to overuse medication may already exist.
5. Cyproheptadine, if used for vascular headache prophylaxis, may produce undesirable weight gain.
6. Weight gain may also occur with prolonged use of tricyclic antidepressants.

Family Counseling

Especially in cases of intractable pain, the support provided by a pain patient's family is often a critical factor in his or her rehabilitation. Family members must learn how to *work with* the patient, reinforcing *normal*—not pain—*behavior.* Family counseling services offered through the pain clinic are intended to bring this important element into concert with other efforts to help patients cope with their problems.

RESEARCH

The puzzling, paradoxical nature of pain remains one of the most challenging *and important* areas in modern health research. An important dimension of any pain clinic's research should be the accumulation and analysis of day-to-day clinical data from which various therapeutic approaches can be evaluated. These studies help to isolate which methods either offer or promise long-term effectiveness, which therapeutic combinations are most successful, etc.

Our own research programs are focused on development of new biofeedback systems as well as evaluation of present approaches, the mechanisms of electrical analgesia (pain-reducing neurostimulation), more accurate objective measurement of pain and evaluation of new, nonnarcotic pain-controlling drugs.

Future research is anticipated to include studies of pain's underlying biologic and physiologic mechanisms.

THE GATE CONTROL THEORY

It is generally agreed that patterning of input is essential to the production of pain. The excessive peripheral stimulation that occurs when one hits one's thumb with a hammer quite obviously evokes pain of an acute nature. In addition, there are specific neural mechanisms that account for the summation of stimuli in clinical situations of chronic pain, in which the provoking stimulus may not be so apparent. Reverberating circuits in spinal internuncial pools may be set off by normally benign afferent input which could thereafter be interpreted centrally as painful. It is proposed that a specialized central system prevents this critical summation from occurring, in that it inhibits synaptic transmission of slowly conducting nerve fibers which ordinarily subserve pain. One must, therefore, evoke the dual concepts of central summation of pain and central inhibition of pain to explain pain as it occurs clinically. Melzack and Wall (1965) modified this theory to propose that the substantia gelatinosa of the dorsal horn of the spinal cord functions as a gate control system which modulates the afferent stimuli before they are transmitted centrally.

Central to the concept of the gate control theory is the substantia gelatinosa, which runs throughout the length of the spinal cord. It is suggested that this area acts as a gate control system modulating the transmission of nerve impulses (Fig. 12.1). Thus, the large myelinated fibers inhibit pain signals, while the small unmyelinated fibers facilitate their transmission. In each case, this is accomplished by the action of the substantia gelatinosa on the spinal cord cells that transmit afferent signals to the brain.

EFFECTS OF ANALGESIC AGENTS

Much information related to the study of pain has been obtained from the study of analgesic agents of varying types. It has been known for some time that receptors in the skin, termed "nociceptors" (responding to tissue-damaging stimuli), have both myelinated and nonmyelinated afferent fibers. Not all nonmyelinated fibers (C-fibers) are specific for nociceptive stimuli, since it has been shown that C-fibers will respond to temperature changes and to mechanical stimuli of only a few milligrams of skin pressure, which do not cause pain. It is important, therefore, to avoid the concept that C-fibers are specific in peripheral nerves for pain. Furthermore, it has been found that fluid obtained from areas where there has been tissue destruction, as in a blister which forms after burning, contains a pain-producing substance which also has vasodilator and vasopermeability-increasing activity. This substance is a vasodilator polypeptide, related to the polypeptide bradykinin. This polypeptide may be a terminal portion of the γ-globulin molecule, from which it can be liberated or separated by proteolytic enzymes. Injury to tissue activates the en-

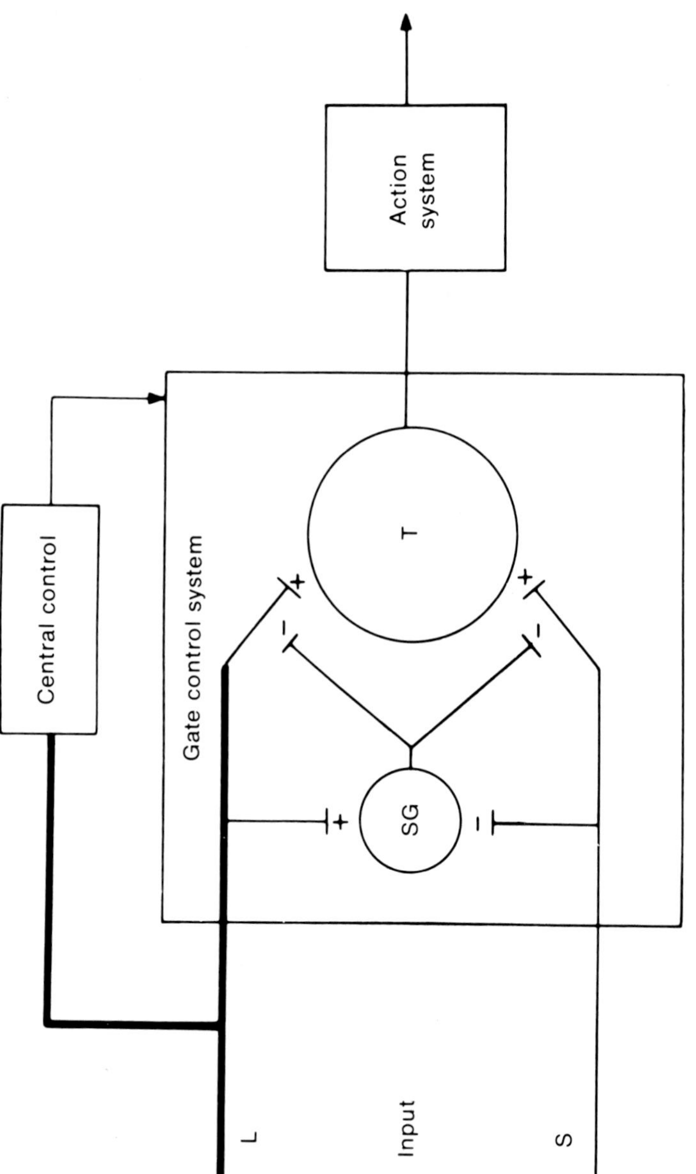

Figure 12.1. Schematic diagram of the gate control theory of pain mechanisms: *L*, the large-diameter fibers; *S*, the small-diameter fibers. The fibers project to the substantia gelatinosa (*SG*) and first central transmission (*T*) cells. The inhibitory effect exerted by *SG* on the afferent fiber terminals is increased by activity in *L* fibers and decreased by activity in *S* fibers. The central control trigger is represented by a line running from the large-fiber system to the central control mechanisms; these mechanisms, in turn, project back to the gate control system. The *T* cells project to the entry cells of the action system. + = excitation, − = inhibitions. (From Melzack R, Wall PD: Pain mechanisms: A new theory. Science 150:971, 1965. Copyright 1965 by the American Association for the Advancement of Science.)

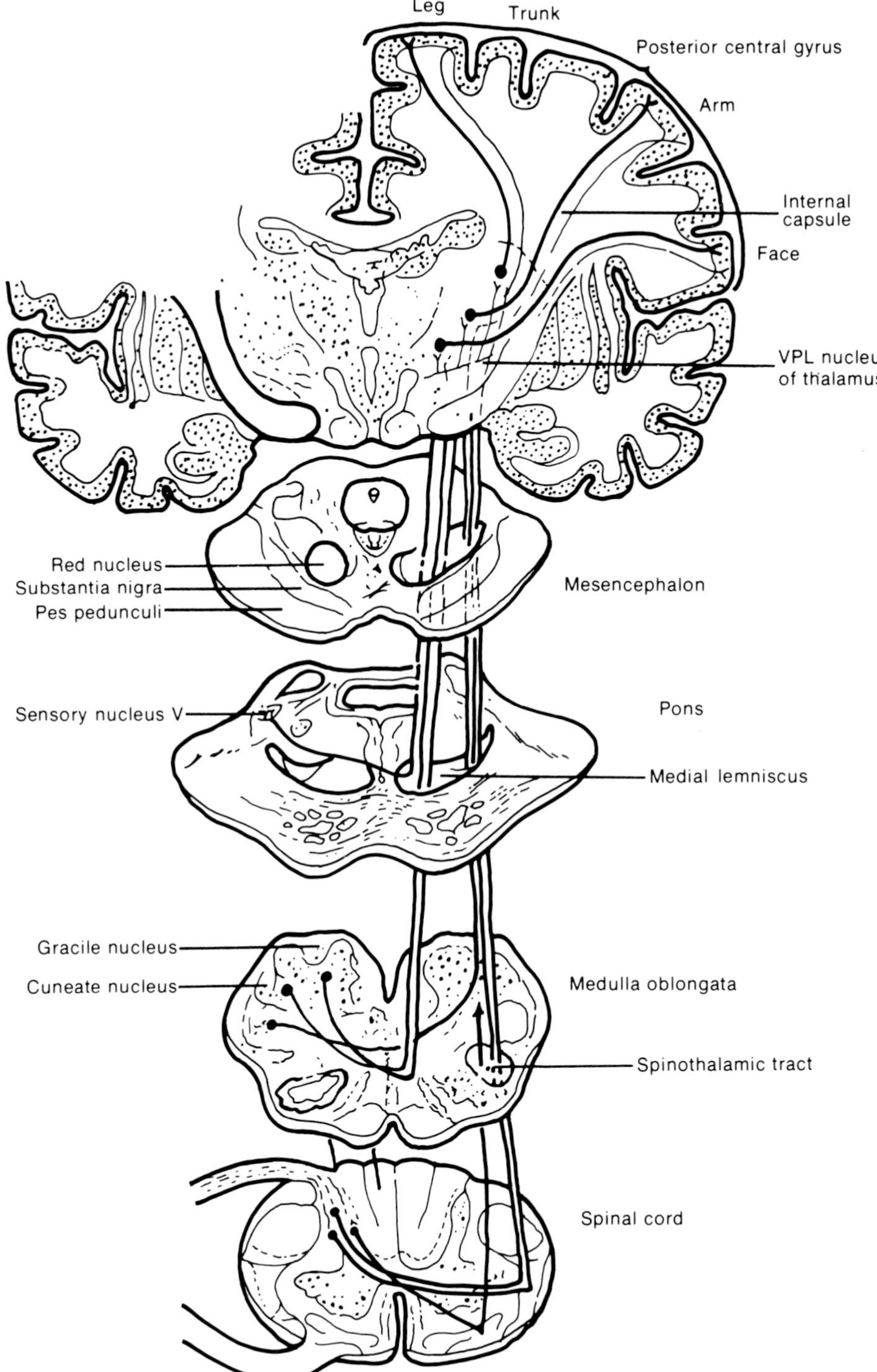

Figure 12.2. A simplified diagram of the main features in the lemniscal somatosensory pathways.

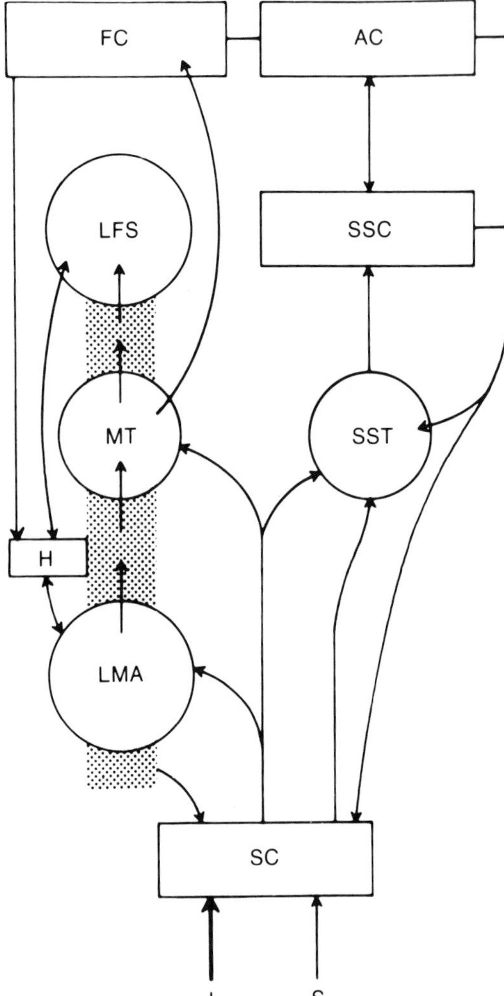

Figure 12.3. Schematic diagram of the anatomic foundation of the proposed pain model. On the right: thalamic and neocortical structures subserving discriminative capacity. On the left: reticular and limbic systems subserving motivational-affective functions. Ascending pathways from the spinal cord (*SC*) are: (1) the dorsal column-lemniscal and dorsolateral tracts (*right ascending arrow*) projecting to the somatosensory thalamus (*SST*) and cortex (*SSC*), and (2) the anterolateral pathways (*left ascending arrow*) to the somatosensory thalamus via the neospinothalamic tract and to the reticular formation (*stripped area*), the limbic midbrain area (*LMA*) and medial thalamus (*MT*) via the paramedial ascending system. Descending pathways to spinal cord originate in somatosensory and associated cortical areas (*AC*) and in the reticular formation. Polysynaptic and reciprocal relationships in limbic and reticular systems are indicated. Other abbreviations: *FC*-frontal cortex; *LFS*-limbic forebrain structures (hippocampus, septum, amygdala, and associated cortex); *H*-hypothalamus. (From Casey K: Toward a neurophysiology of pain. Headache 8:141, 1969.)

zymes which lead to the formation of bradykinin. Prostaglandins are also liberated. Salicylates, such as aspirin and related compounds, exert a peripheral analgesic effect by interfering with the actions of the kinins and by inhibiting prostaglandin synthesis.

Wolff et al. (1960) have demonstrated that antidromic dorsal root activity plays some role in the liberation of vasodilator polypeptides of the bradykinin type. They suggest that neurogenically induced vasodilation may represent a direct contribution of the nervous system to the inflammatory reaction. Interactions within the spinal cord may play a role in the central perception of pain. The flexor response in man is studied by recording electromyographically the response in the vastus medialis muscle when pain stimuli have been applied at different skin territories of the same limb. The flexor reflex consists of the contraction of the limb at the ankle, knee and hip, when noxious stimulation is applied, in order to withdraw the limb from the site of noxious stimulation. This is an integrated and organized reflex, which serves as a withdrawal response. Under hypnotic analgesia, inhibition is evoked and no excitatory activity follows. This illustrates that painful flexor reflexes in man are subject to modulation from higher centers.

Chapman et al. (1960) demonstrated changes in tissue vulnerability induced during hypnotic suggestion. Following standard amounts of noxious stimulation of the forearm during hypnosis, decreased inflammatory reaction and tissue damage were observed when the suggestion was made that the arm was insensitive and numb, as compared with the reaction and tissue damage of the other arm which was suggested to be normally sensitive. When the suggestion was made that the forearm was tender, increased inflammatory reaction and tissue damage were observed, as compared with the normally sensitive arm. On the basis of these studies it is postulated that neural activity can alter inflammatory reactions in peripheral tissues.

Postulation: Neural activity can alter inflammatory reactions in peripheral tissue.

Narcotics exert a suppressive action on spinal reflexes, probably by augmenting supraspinal inhibition of cord reflexes. Reflex suppression by morphine is greater when the spinal cord is intact than when it is transected. Spinal cord reflexes can also be diminished by the use of medications which are not analgesics in the usual sense, especially anticonvulsants. Studies on the use of the anticonvulsant carbamazepine in tic douloureux suggest that inhibition of spinal cord reflex activity may provide analgesia. Thus, tic douloureux, an extremely unpleasant pain syndrome, may be manifested by a state of abnormal reactivity of the spinal trigeminal nuclei, related to a decreased or defective central integrative system regulating sensory input. Tic douloureux has been proposed as a model for this type of syndrome, wherein the inability of the brain to suppress sensory input from normal or minimally damaged peripheral tissues evokes severe pain.

THE BRAIN'S FUNCTION

This latter proposition of pain related to abnormal spinal reflex activity leads naturally to considerations of central handling of pain in the brain. Here the dual functions in the somatosensory system of man should be emphasized. One component of this system is represented by the lemniscal system, which is a precise, topographic system of somatic sensation involving the peripheral nerves, the first order afferent fibers of the dorsal columns of the spinal cord, the neural elements of the medial lemniscus, and the cells of the ventrobasal nuclear complex of the thalamus and of the post central region of the cerebral cortex (Fig. 12.2). A second, phylogenetically older system, designated the anterolateral system, originates in the dorsal horn of the spinal cord.

In contrast, the anterolateral system is poorly defined and ascends in nonlinear tracts to multiple areas of the brain, including the thalamus, midbrain, medulla, and especially the reticular system and the limbic system. The anterolateral system is hard to illustrate in a precise neuroanatomic way but is pictured schematically in Figure 12.3.

The neurons in this latter pathway have properties different from those in the lemniscal system. Their receptive fields are very large and not topographically organized and often lack specificity. Medications such as narcotics exert their effects primarily on the anterolateral projection system and thus produce diffuse pain-alleviating effects. There are other experimental studies in animals which support this concept—that is, that the lemniscal and anterolateral systems differ in their pharmacologic reactivity. Melzack produced neural responses by stimulating the tooth pulp of cats; these neural responses appeared both in the lemniscal and in the anterolateral systems. It was shown in these experiments that nitrous oxide selectively abolished the response from the lemniscal system only. These pharmacologic differences may relate to differences in the size of the fiber tracts rather than to those in the number of associated synapses (Fig. 12.4).

Antidepressants of the tricyclic type have been employed in the management of chronic pain syndromes, especially headache. These agents may decrease pain by altering central appreciation of the quality or intensity of pain as it occurs in the depressed patient. As a consequence of his depression, the depressed patient may misinterpret afferent stimuli at the cortical level and may experience pain when, in fact, he should not. The structural relationship of the tricyclic antidepressants to anticonvulsants such as carbamazepine is striking. It is important to realize

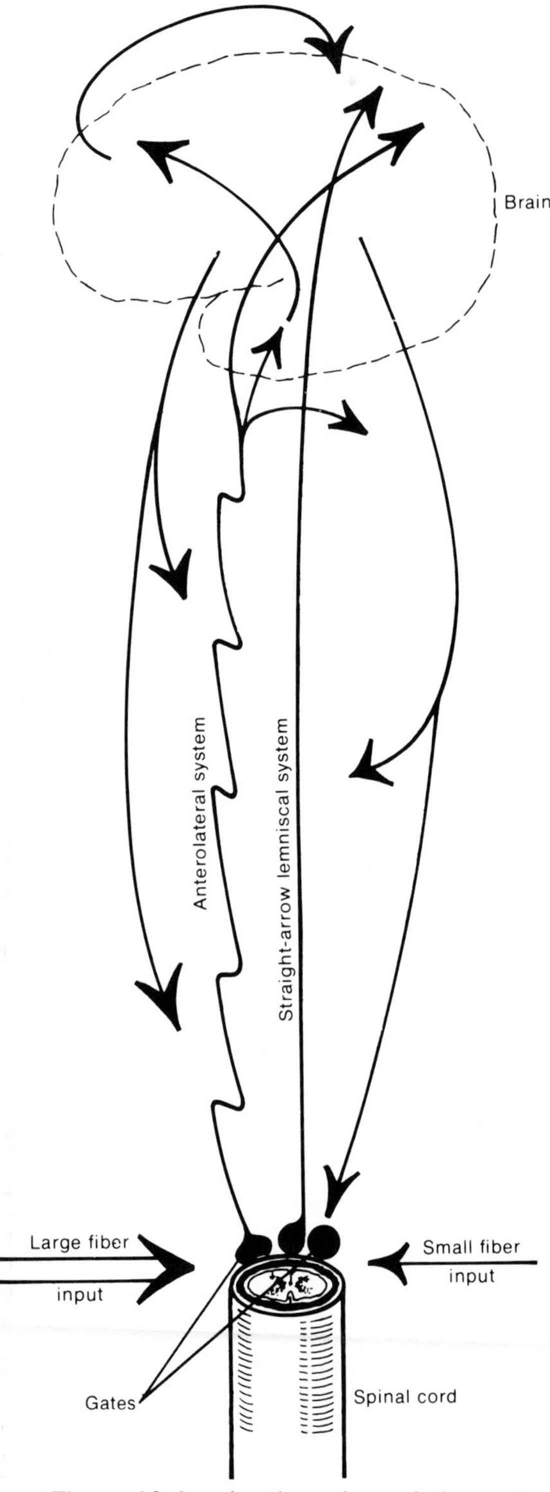

Figure 12.4. Another view of the gate control system.

that the anterolateral system projects especially to those areas of the brain which have to do with basic behavioral mechanisms, with personality and with motivation and affect, and all of these aspects of central nervous activities strongly influence pain perception.

The depressed patient may misinterpret afferent stimuli and experience pain when, in fact, he should not.

The brain itself exerts significant control over information it receives. Probably a portion of the brainstem reticular formation exerts a tonic inhibitory influence on information transmission. This may occur not only at the spinal gate but also at any other synaptic level at which sensory information is projected rostrally. Thus, the gate control theory is also compatible with the clinical experience that pain can be intensified or decreased by psychologic factors. Just as in biofeedback experiments, in which there is brain control over sensory input, so methods of conditioning may be employed in situations of chronic pain. In cases of chronic headache, for example, in which a chronic pain cycle has been produced, it should be possible, using methods of relaxation, suggestion, biofeedback control, and, possibly, hypnosis, to reduce pain perception through cortical activity, which acts to increase inhibition at the spinal gate and other synaptic levels.

Thus, what we are saying in so many words is that the brain itself can modify and change painful stimuli, and it can do this is at least two ways (Fig. 12.5).

1. Peripherally, by closing the spinal gate and not letting the stimulus into the spinal cord
2. Centrally, by modifying ongoing central nervous activity

Thus it may be seen that pain is an integrated experience which is dependent upon

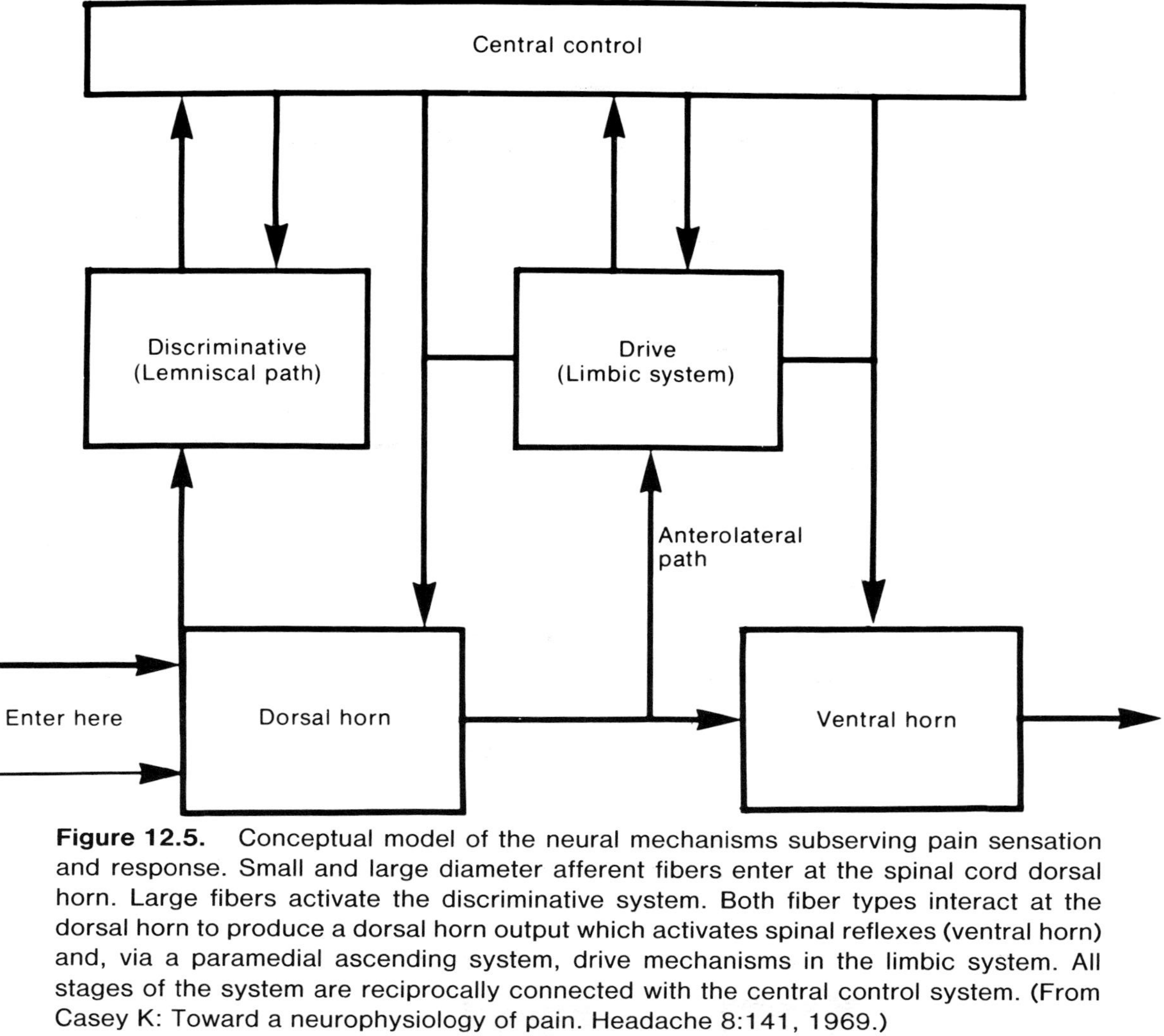

Figure 12.5. Conceptual model of the neural mechanisms subserving pain sensation and response. Small and large diameter afferent fibers enter at the spinal cord dorsal horn. Large fibers activate the discriminative system. Both fiber types interact at the dorsal horn to produce a dorsal horn output which activates spinal reflexes (ventral horn) and, via a paramedial ascending system, drive mechanisms in the limbic system. All stages of the system are reciprocally connected with the central control system. (From Casey K: Toward a neurophysiology of pain. Headache 8:141, 1969.)

an intact and functioning central nervous system, involving the peripheral nerves, the spinal cord and the brain. Psychologic factors such as past experience, attention and emotion may influence pain response and perception greatly. It is to be emphasized that the quantitative measurement of pain is hazardous, that pain is an individual perception which the perceiver may communicate only poorly, and that laboratory models of experimental pain may be difficult to interpret, especially in terms of clinical situations wherein analgesia is sought.

MEASURING PAIN SEVERITY

Sternbach et al. (1974) have shown that it is possible to relate the patient's pain estimate to a tourniquet pain ratio in an attempt to more adequately measure the amount of suffering the patient is experiencing. This measurement is important not only in making a correct diagnosis but also in deciding to what extent medical and/or surgical procedures may be necessary to relieve the pain. If one relies solely on the patient's description of the intensity of the pain, one invites error from other factors, particularly personality variables and cultural differences in pain appreciation.

The pain estimate is obtained by asking the patient to rate the intensity of his/her pain on a scale of 0–100. Zero represents no pain at all, and 100 is pain so severe that one would commit suicide if it had to be endured. The patient frequently estimates the pain daily at the same time that activity management in terms of hours up and out of bed is calculated. In addition, the tourniquet pain ratio can be obtained using an ischemic test developed by Smith, which makes use of partial ischemia of the arm associated with exercise. (See Tourniquet Pain Test Procedures.) Neither the pain estimate nor the tourniquet pain ratio seem to be correlated with any clinical personality variable on the Minnesota Multiphasic Personality Inventory (MMPI) or on a Health Index, but the pain estimate is usually higher than the tourniquet pain ratio, presumably due to a mixture of pain perception and communication needs.

Tourniquet Pain Test

Procedures

1. Have patient lie down.
2. Identify which is nondominant arm (opposite from one used for writing). Ask patient if there is anything wrong with that arm. If the nondominant arm is o.k., it will be used for the test on each occasion. Otherwise, the dominant arm should be used.
3. Have patient remove any jewelry (watch, rings, etc.) from arm to be used.
4. Explain the basic procedure to the patient in a brief fashion and mention that he may ask questions if he wishes.
5. Raise the arm to be used and then begin wrapping arm with rubber Esmarch bandage. Wrap the arm very tightly, starting with the top of the finger tips to just slightly beyond the elbow. Tuck any extra bandage roll into the wrappings.
6. Inflate blood pressure cuff to 250, with the cuff placed in the normal position, and just at the end of the Esmarch bandage.
7. Remove Esmarch bandage.
8. Lower arm and begin stop watch for a 60-second pause. During this period, make sure the cuff stays at 250.
9. Give patient hand exerciser and tell him to squeeze-release, every 2 seconds for 20 squeezes. When second hand passes 1 minute 20 seconds, he will have completed 20 squeezes.
10. *Restart* stop watch by pressing side button. Timing begins when last squeeze completed.
11. Ask patient to tell when what he feels in his arm feels similar to: (a) the average pain he has had for the past week; (b) the "unbearable" level (the most he can take).

12. When patient says the pain in his arm is unbearable, stop the watch by pressing the large center knob and release the cuff. That is the end of the test.

NOTE: Be sure patient compares arm feeling to pain he has had. Question him if he says it is "unbearable" and has not mentioned clinical pain.

If patient does not reach "clinical" level in 15 minutes, stop the test and remove cuff.

Compute ratio: $\frac{\text{Clinical pain level}}{\text{Maximum tolerance}}$ $\times 100$;

Example: $\frac{\text{3 min, 10 sec}}{\text{5 min, 40 sec}} = \frac{190}{340} = 56\%$

Instructions to Patients

(Read or repeat to patients on their first testing.)

We're going to do an experiment to test your pain thresholds, to help the doctors understand the level of pain you feel.

I will first wrap your arm tightly with this rubber bandage. Then, I'll inflate a blood pressure cuff on your arm, and then have you squeeze a hand exerciser 20 times. This is in order to drain the blood from the veins in your arm as much as possible.

Then you will just lay your arm down, and then I want you to tell me when what you feel in your arm equals the pain which you have had for the past week. It may be a different kind of pain, but when the severity is the same, or it hurts as much, let me know.

Then, I want you to tell me when what you feel in your arm is unbearable. When you tell me it is unbearable, that you cannot take any more, I will take the cuff off and the test will be over.

Remember, I want you to tell me when the level of pain in your arm equals your clinical pain.

Please don't move or talk during the test. Do you have any questions?

MORPHINE, OPIATE RECEPTORS, ENKEPHALINS AND PITUITARY ENDORPHINS

Morphine and its derivatives exert their effects by binding to specific receptor sites on cells in the brain and spinal cord. Morphine-like substances which occur naturally in the body may also act at those sites. Opiate receptors in the brain have been identified by measuring the specific binding of radioactively labeled opiate drugs to cell fragments from different brain areas. Much the largest amount of binding was found in cells of the limbic system. This suggests that the opiates exert their analgesic and euphoria-producing effects by binding to receptors in the limbic system.

Optical isomers of the opiate analgesics have different pharmacologic activities. Only the levorotatory isomer produces the characteristic analgesic effects of the drug. The dextrorotatory isomer is totally inactive. This stereospecificity of opiate actions supports the model of a highly specific receptor which can recognize the mirror image form of the opiate molecule.

Opiate antagonists are substances that specifically block the analgesic and euphoric actions of opiates without eliciting any such effects themselves. These antagonists are opiates which are transformed by very slight molecular modifications into antagonists. It seems likely that opiate antagonists will occupy opiate receptor sites, are inert themselves, but prevent the opiates from reaching the receptor sites and in this manner inhibit analgesia and euphoria.

The opiates are also of interest with respect to the two major brain pathways implicated in the perception of pain. Opiates are considerably more effective in interfering with dull, chronic and less-localized pain which is transmitted to the central nervous system through the paleospinothalamic pathway. Sharp and well-localized pain, transmitted through the lemniscal system, responds more poorly to opiates. If one maps the distribution of opiate receptors in the brain, one finds that they parallel in a striking fashion the paleospinothalamic pathway. Similarly, spinal cord opiate receptors can be localized in the area about the substantia gelatinosa, which, as discussed before, is a way station for the brainward conduction of sensory information associated with pain.

Since specific opiate receptors are a characteristic of most animals and man, the speculation arose that a natural neurotransmitter, morphine-like, would be found in the brain, acting at opiate receptors. In a series of brilliant studies, Hughes (1975), Kosterlitz, Pasternak and Snyder (1978) were able to isolate a morphine-like factor from the brains of animals, particularly pigs, and found that it consisted of two closely related peptides made up of five amino acid units. The term "enkephalin" was given to these peptides. Accumulated evidence suggests that the enkephalins are neurotransmitters of specific neuronal systems in the brain which mediate information having to do with pain and emotional behavior. Furthermore, enkephalin brain levels tend to parallel the distribution of opiate receptors.

The enkephalins work by inhibiting the polarization of brain cells by excitatory transmitters. In effect, enkephalin will mimic morphine to the extent that the inhibition of enkephalin, like that of morphine, is blocked by the opiate antagonist naxolone. This suggests that both morphine and enkephalin act at the same receptor. The relationship between enkephalins and morphine has led to suggestions that the naturally occurring enkephalins may be important in the production of physical addiction.

Even more recently, Goldstein and Li have discovered that natural opiate-like peptides are contained in the pituitary gland (1976). Li has named these peptides "endorphins" for endogenous morphine. These have a high degree of analgesic activity and again are directly blocked by naloxone, a specific opiate antagonist. Guillemin of the Salk Institute has isolated several other peptides from a mixture of hypothalamus and pituitary tissue of pigs (1977). The function of the pituitary endorphins is uncertain, but they may regulate pituitary functions which are known to be altered by opiates, such as the release of the antidiuretic hormone from the posterior pituitary by morphine.

Some of the naturally occurring "internal opiates" have been demonstrated to produce catatonia and other signs of psychiatric disturbance, leading to the further supposition that they may be implicated in various forms of mental illness. Clearly, the discovery of the opiate receptors and their internal opiates is one of the most exciting developments in neurochemistry in recent years. Their relationship to chronic pain states, to addiction, and possibly to basic forms of mental disease will be of concern to all physicians for the foreseeable future.

THE CONCEPT OF SOMATIZATION

The term "somatization" is an abstract one which has several meanings. It refers to the physiological expression of emotions such as anxiety, resentment, depression, etc. Thus, the sweaty palms and tachycardia in anxiety, the gastric hyperactivity and increase in diastolic blood pressure in suppressed anger, and the psychomotor retardation and early morning awakening in depression are examples of somatization. In physiological terms, these responses define the disorders. In psychological terms, they "express" the affective disturbance. Such diseases as cardiac arrhythmias, duodenal ulcers, and essential or labile hypertension are referred to as somatization ("psychosomatic") disorders.

Somatization also includes the concept of psychogenic disorders of physical function, such as blindness, paralysis, deafness, or pain, formerly labeled "conversion" symptoms. Although in former times a distinction was made between psychophysiological disorders (which primarily involved the autonomic nervous system) and conversion disorders (which primarily involved the voluntary nervous system and special senses), such distinctions were often blurred in clinical cases. Thus the term "somatization"—the physical expression of an emotional or psychological disorder—directs attention to that which is being expressed (Sternbach, 1974).

Whatever the emotion or stress response or psychological conflict, the somatization process serves the function of masking the problem from the patient's awareness. This is in contrast to the "professional" psychiatric patient who wallows miserably in subjective distress, analyzing his neurosis in interminable psychotherapy. The somatizer, on the other hand, frequently denies any mood disturbance and is only dimly aware of any problem or stress in his life (Pilowsky, 1978).

From this description, it is apparent that headache patients are very like somatizers. Indeed, one of the complications of diagnosis and treatment is the fact that it is sometimes difficult to assign proper weight to psychological and physical contributions to the pain symptom. This is because, once a pain associated with tissue damage has occurred and becomes chronic, it becomes a "sink" for all intrapsychic and interpersonal stresses and problems. The patient can now become oblivious to familial and occupational sources of tension, can gratify dependency needs by adoption of the sick role, and can have a legitimate source of narcotics, etc.

These considerations suggest the terms "functional overlay" or "secondary gains" of former years, but such terms fail to convey the primacy of mechanisms involved. It has been suggested that one useful solution to the problem of terminology is to emphasize the behavior involved (Fordyce, 1976). All pain behavior is either respondent (Pavlovian) or operant (Skinnerian) in nature—the former reflexive, the latter maintained by environmental reinforcers. This also then suggests the possibility of an analysis leading to appropriate treatment (Fordyce, 1978).

EVERYTHING YOU ALWAYS WANTED TO KNOW ABOUT ACUPUNCTURE

Question: Just exactly what is acupuncture?

Answer: Acupuncture is a method of treatment several thousand years old, which has been used by the Chinese in curing disease and protecting health. In primitive society, acupuncture was administered with a piece of sharp stone called a "pien." A cure was effected by pressing or pricking a certain section of the body. Later the pien was replaced by needles made of stone, bone or bamboo. After metals were discovered, copper, iron and silver needles were used. Modern acupuncture is performed with fine needles of stainless steel.

Q: What is the basis of classical acupuncture?

A: This is related to the ancient Chinese theory that a balance of two forces, the yin and the yang, exists in the universe—and in the human body. The yin represents negative forces of darkness, femaleness, cold and passivity, while yang represents the positives of light, maleness, heat and activity. A disease may result when there is an imbalance of the yin and the yang, which disrupts the orderly flow of life energy through the body. According to this theory, the major body organs, 12 in all, are divided between the yin and the yang. The yin organs include the liver, spleen and heart, while the gallbladder, large intestine and stomach are yang organs. Life energy is said to flow from organ to organ through a network of channels beneath the skin, termed "meridians." There are 12 meridians, representing the organs, running on either side of the body, with two extra meridians, one along the center in the front of the body and one in the back. In addition, the network of meridians contains 500 to 800 points which the acupuncturist must learn in order to correctly place his needles and "correct the energy flow and balances." These points are quite specific. One point on the hand, for example, is for toothaches, sore throat and anesthesia. One point on the leg is for stomachache and appendicitis. A point on the foot is used for treating ulcers, fever, coughing and so on. Manual manipulation or heating of the acupuncture needle may be incorporated into this treatment.

Q: What is acupuncture anesthesia?

A: In acupuncture anesthesia, one or more needles are inserted at certain points on the patient's limbs, ears, nose or face. Anesthesia follows after a period of inducement or stimulation, often one-half hour, and then the operation is performed. Patients are fully conscious during operations when this kind of anesthesia is used. They may receive some preanesthetic medications, but the amount and type of preanesthetic medication are not usually emphasized in Chinese publications on the subject. Evidently there are many patients who receive no preanesthetic medication. In some situations during acupuncture anesthesia, electrical stimulation of the needles is necessary to achieve pain relief.

Q: How many patients have received this type of acupuncture anesthesia?

A: The Chinese claim that more than

400,000 patients, including children and people in their 80s, have received acupuncture anesthesia for surgical operations. They claim a success rate of 90%. Operations have included procedures on the brain, removal of the lung and even correction of congenital cardiac defects. Acupuncture anesthesia does not need complicated apparatus and is applicable regardless of equipment, climate and geographical conditions. It can, therefore, be widely used in the cities and is particularly suitable to mountainous and rural areas and under conditions of war.

Q: What sort of knowledge is required to use acupuncture anesthesia?

A: So far as can be determined, acupuncture anesthesia can be learned quickly and does not require elaborate professional instruction. Chinese publications show medical workers experimenting on each other, placing needles in order to locate the most effective points for producing anesthesia.

The Chinese use acupuncture for a whole series of medical problems related to pain.

Q: Is acupuncture helpful in medical conditions?

A: The Chinese use acupuncture for a whole series of medical problems related to pain. These include especially arthritis, headache (including migraine) and hypertension. The Chinese make great claims for treatment of eye diseases with acupuncture, including glaucoma and even blindness. It should be recognized that Chinese physicians do not believe in rigidly controlled studies, and some of the claims for treatment of medical diseases particularly should be viewed with great scepticism. There is no question, however, that in some situations acupuncture works.

Q: Is acupuncture anesthesia a new concept?

A: According to Chinese publications, this form of anesthesia is a direct result of the teachings of Chairman Mao who pointed out that "Chinese medicine and pharmacology are a great treasure-house; efforts should be made to explore them and raise them to a higher level." In responding to this call in the 1950s, Chinese medical workers developed a "revolutionary spirit" and applied modern scientific knowledge and methods to acupuncture. It is of interest that the entire story of acupuncture anesthesia as described by the Chinese is full of political implications. For example, it is stated in a book on acupuncture anesthesia produced by the Foreign Languages Press of Peking, in 1972, that "no sooner had acupuncture anesthesia appeared than it was repressed by Liu Shao Chi's counterrevolutionary revisionist line and attacked by bourgeois experts. In a vain attempt to nip it in the bud, they raved that it was not scientific, without any practical value, and a retrogression in the history of anesthesia."

It is further stated that "the great proletarian cultural revolution swept away the bourgeois trash, and revolutionary medical workers relentlessly criticized Liu Shao Chi's counterrevolutionary revisionist line and work in scientific research. This facilitated great development in improvement in acupuncture anesthesia." Political diatribes such as this, which appear in the discussion of a scientific method of anesthesia, make Western observers critical of acupuncture and of Chinese studies of its efficacy.

Q: Is acupuncture anesthesia invariably effective?

A: Even the Chinese admit that it may still have "some imperfections." They admit that at certain stages in some operations patients still "feel some pain" and "some feel uncomfortable when the internal organs are pulled." They further state that "Chinese medical and scientific workers are making still greater efforts in studying Marxism-Leninism-Mao Tse Tung thought and are using dialectical materialism to guide their medical work in scientific research. Daring in practice and in breaking new ground, they are bending their efforts to perfect acupuncture anesthesia."

Q: How might acupuncture anesthesia work?

A: Surprisingly, there are few suggestions in Chinese writings which indicate the mechanism by which acupuncture anesthesia works, and there is apparently little interest in this subject. The explanation for acupuncture, on a scientific basis, has come by and large from Western medicine. It has been known for years that stimulation of the skin tends to reduce pain, related primarily to the speed of conduction of pain sensations as related to those of touch. Sensations of touch are conducted along the nerves at a much more rapid rate than are those of pain. It is theoretically possible, therefore, to block out sensations of pain by producing simultaneous stimulation of the skin. We all know this well. For example, when a child falls down, his mother advises him to rub the uninjured area around the skin abrasion and, frequently, this reduces the pain. Grandmother produced the same effect with her mustard plasters and, even now, irritating rubs are sold to reduce muscle pain. Presumably these act by producing counterirritation and stimulation of the skin and thereby block out the pain from the aching muscles. This concept—of a gate control mechanism regulating pain—was first formulated by Melzack and Wall (1965), who proposed that a specific area of the spinal cord functions as a gate that modulates the amount of stimuli that is allowed to flow into the spinal cord and eventually to the conscious brain.

Recent studies have suggested that acupuncture alleviates pain by stimulating production of endogenous opiates. Pomeranz and Paley (1979) of the University of Toronto discovered that the opiate antogonist naloxone blocked acupuncture anesthesia in mice and cited other studies in which naloxone had not blocked hypnosis-induced analgesia in humans.

Q: Can acupuncture anesthesia be considered a form of hypnosis?

A: There is no question that some aspect of hypnosis play a role in acupuncture anesthesia, but it is unlikely that the entire explanation for acupuncture anesthesia can be related to hypnotic effects. Operations under hypnosis are effective in perhaps 10–20% of patients. Operations under acupuncture have a considerably higher success rate, approaching 90% effectiveness in some areas, such as surgery of the thyroid. Although conditions in China may lead to a greater acceptance and confidence in the mystique of acupuncture, as representing a method of anesthesia officially approved by the government, it seems unwise to use to assume that the beneficial effects of acupuncture anesthesia are entirely related to a hypnotic trance effective in a particular cultural milieu.

Q: In other words, acupuncture anesthesia probably has a neurophysiologic basis?

A: Correct. Whether it is related to the gating effect mentioned above, to an increase in cortical inhibition of afferent input, to alteration in postsynaptic inhibition of impulses, to spreading depression of the sensory cortex itself or to modulation by the endogenous opiates (all of which have been suggested as possible explanations) is currently moot. Obviously this method of anesthesia requires further study.

Q: Would acupuncture anesthesia be an improvement over modern anesthetic techniques?

A: Although it is obvious that modern anesthetic techniques should not be abandoned, there are certain aspects of acupuncture anesthesia which deserve serious consideration. Anesthesia by acupuncture helps to prevent disorders of the patient's physiologic functions during surgery and avoids the harmful side effects of the use of anesthesia after its completion. The patient's blood pressure, pulse and breathing in general remain normal. Incisions tend to heal more quickly and functions of the internal organs are restored quickly and more satisfactorily after the operation, as a consequence of which the patient can move about and take food early. Acupuncture may have its particular application in patients who are poor operative risks because of poor functioning of the liver, kidneys or lungs, in whom administration of anesthesia by drugs is not advisable. Certainly it promotes early ambulation, a goal of Western anesthetic practices as well.

References

Casey K (1969) Toward a neurophysiology of pain. *Headache 8:*141.

Chapman LF, Ramos AL, Goodell H, et al. (1960) Neurokinin: A polypeptide formed during neuronal activity in man. *Trans Am Neurol Assoc 85:*42.

Dalessio DJ (1980) *Wolff's Headache and Other Head*

Pain, ed 4. New York, Oxford University Press.
Fordyce, WE (1976) *Behavioral Methods for Chronic Pain and Illness.* CV Mosby, St. Louis.
Fordyce WE (1978) Learning processes in pain. In *The Psychology of Pain*, edited by Sternbach RA. New York, Raven Press, p. 49.
Goldstein A (1976) Opioid peptides (endorphins) in pituitary and brain. *Science 193:*1081–1086.
Guillemin R (1977) Endorphins, brain peptides that act like opiates. *N Engl J Med 296:*226–228.
Hughes J, Smith TW, Kosterlitz LA, et al. Identification of two related pentapeptides from the brain with potent opiate agonist activity. *Nature 258:*577–579.
Melzak R, Wall PD (1965) Pain mechanisms: A new theory. *Science 150:*971–979.
Pilowsky I (1978) Psychodynamic aspects of the pain experience. In *The Psychology of Pain*, edited by Sternbach RA. New York, Raven Press, p. 203.
Pomeranz B, Paley D (1979) Electroacupuncture hypalgesia is mediated by afferent nerve impulses: An electrophysiological study in mice. *Exp Neurol 66:*398–402.
Smith GM, Lowenstein E, Hubbard JH, et al. (1967) Experimental pain produced by the submaximum effort tourniquet technique: Further evidence of validity. *J Pharmacol Exp Ther 163:*468.
Snyder SH (1978) The opiate receptor and morphine-like peptides in the brain. *Am J Psychiatry 135:*645–652.
Sternbach RA (1974) *Pain Patients: Traits and Treatment.* New York, Academic Press.
Sternbach RA, Murphy RW, Timmermans G, Greenhoot JH, Akeson WH (1974) Measuring the severity of clinical pain. In *Advances in Neurology*, vol 4, *International Symposium on Pain*, edited by Bonica JJ. New York, Raven Press, pp. 281–288.
Wolff HG (1963) *Headache and Other Head Pain.* New York, Oxford University Press.

work too hard at the exercises.) They may imagine putting their hands in a tub of hot water or sitting on a hot beach or by a fire. They are also told to focus on a relaxing image, like being on a rubber mattress in a pool with the sunlight streaming down on their hands. We have also found that it is very helpful for the patient to listen to a tape of the autogenic phrases while on the monitor. Success at training has been particularly demonstrated when the patient listens to his own voice reading the phrases since they sometimes tend to resist training when listening to a tape in the clinician's voice.

HOME PRACTICE

As mentioned, the techniques just described are sufficiently learned only with diligent home practice by the patient. All patients are given detailed instructions to accomplish this.

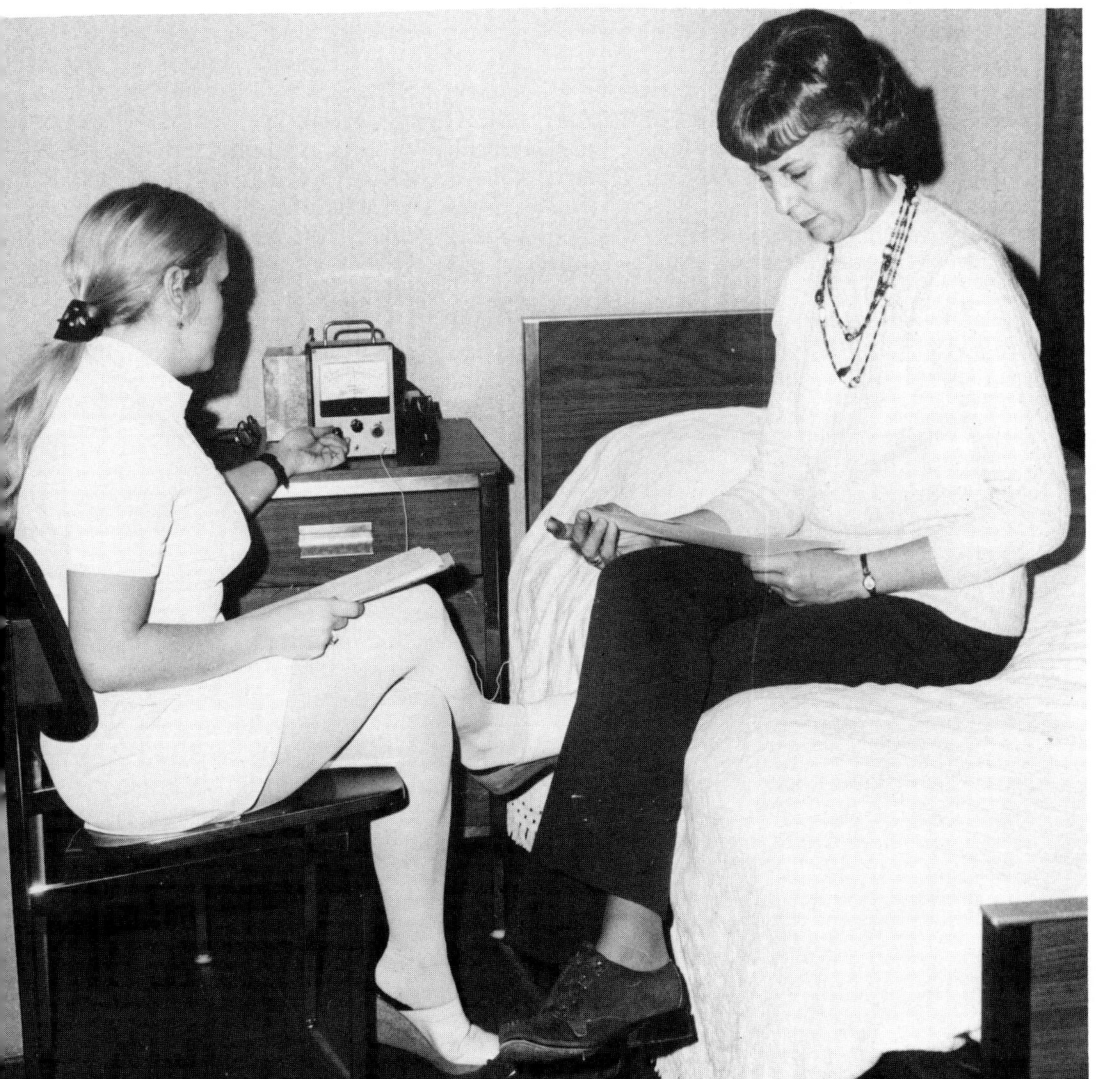

Figure 13.4. Autogenic trainer teaches patient to raise temperature in the hands.

A temperature biofeedback monitor is provided on a rental basis for at least the first 4 weeks of therapy, as an integral part of the home training program. In addition to the monitor, the patient is also provided with either a list or a tape of autogenic phrases to be used in conjunction with the biofeedback as is done in the Clinic.

Patients are instructed to use their home trainer twice daily, for 10–15 minutes each session. They are also encouraged to employ it with their emerging control skills whenever preheadache warnings occur, or at the time of headache onset. The importance of twice daily practice must be stressed at this point. The patient is told repeatedly that in this way he builds the very self-control skills which decrease the chance of his experiencing a headache. Since many patients experience early awakening due to headaches or wake up in the morning with a headache already present, they are also instructed to practice immediately before bedtime.

Each patient with a temperature feedback monitor at home is encouraged to keep a daily diary and record what occurs during all practice sessions. The patient should first record the degree of warmth at the pretraining session. If he is aware of his hands being quite warm before he starts to practice, he should not be discouraged by a small increase in temperature during the session, as he began in a state of substantial vasodilation. At the end of each session, patients should record their degree of relaxation as well as possible change of mood during the session. If patients concentrate too hard, they may experience post session tension. This should all be recorded, as well as the exact amount of change in the hand temperature during the session, in degrees.

After the first week of training, the patients should begin to record the speed at which they achieve warmth. This is important as the patient may need only a 2- or 3-degree change in temperature to successfully abort a migraine. If this can be accomplished in 1 or 2 minutes, the patient may be able to use his new skill effectively at the first signs of a headache. The patient should try to elevate his hand temperature 1 degree in 1 minute. When this has been achieved, the goal should be increased to 1½ degrees and increased thereafter, assuming, of course, that each goal has been achieved.

EMG FEEDBACK TRAINING

Following each in-clinic temperature training session, an electromyographic session is administered (Fig. 13.5). The EMG trainer is used exclusively in the office. Patients make two or three Clinic visits per week during the first month, with the visits gradually decreasing from then on. Out-of-town patients receive more intensive training and are seen twice daily for 2 weeks. To record the patient's progress, a daily chart is kept, noting frequency, severity and duration of headaches.

The sessions generally last 20 minutes and are conducted in a dark, quiet room, immediately following the temperature session. The patient remains in a reclining position and is told that we are monitoring frontalis muscle activity and that if facial, shoulder and/or neck muscles are tense a high-pitched tone is produced. It is suggested that he focus on relaxation of the entire body while receiving biofeedback. As relaxation is achieved, the pitch of the tone decreases. The patient is advised to experiment with positions, moving around in the chair until maximum relaxation is achieved.

Electrodes are placed on each temple and a set of stereo headphones is used to minimize external distractions. The EMG monitor is equipped with variable sensitivities so that, as the patient reduces tension at one level, the monitor can be reset to the next higher sensitivity. With each level, decreasing the tone becomes more challenging.

As with temperature training, instructions are used to assist the patient in discovering how to relax the frontalis muscles and the other target muscles just described. The patient must learn to identify certain tensor points in his facial, neck and shoulder areas, while using the biofeedback monitor. In order to aid the patient in this task, certain progressive relaxation exercises adapted from the work of Wolpe are given to the patient (Fig. 13.6). These exercises should be practiced at home twice daily, without biofeedback instrumentation. If the patient is using the temperature trainer also, then the EMG exercises should be done second. There is a tendency for the hands to become warmer during progressive relaxation exercises, thereby diminishing the effect of the hand-warming procedures. As with temperature control, many patients have noted a decrease in the severity of their headaches when they practice the progressive relaxation exercises at the first symptoms of a headache.

Home use of these exercises and clinical sessions on the EMG monitor assist the patient in recognizing stress points. Common stress points often identified by patients include: teeth grinding, jaw clenching, tightening of the forehead, wrinkling of the brow, obvious tension in the neck and tightening of the shoulders. By learning to relax these points in times of stress, at the first symptoms of headache, and at bedtime, patients have noticed a reduction in the severity of their headaches. Patients who are diligent in practicing the temperature and EMG exercises will usually experience a decrease in the frequency of their headaches as well. A common occurrence is the patient who experiences a decrease in the frequency of migraine headaches and an increase in the milder muscle contraction headache. What seems to be happening, in reality, is that the more severe migraine has masked the muscle contraction headache, and when the migraine disappears the milder form draws more attention. These too will eventually disappear with continued practice of the temperature and EMG exercises.

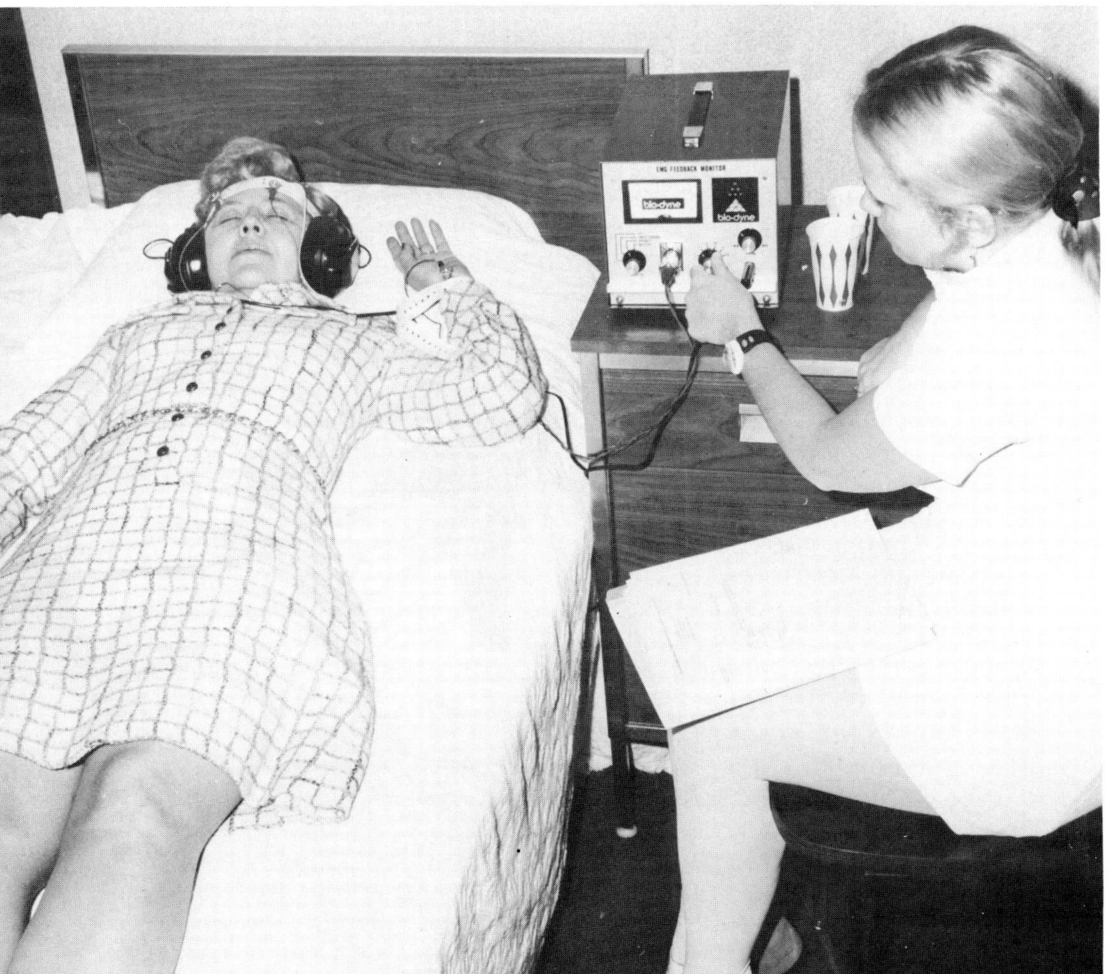

Figure 13.5. Patient learns to relax by means of electromyographic biofeedback.

THE THERAPIST

It must be emphasized that in the biofeedback training program the role of the therapist, or the technician, is a focal one. On the first visit the therapist explains the goals of biofeedback training. Current articles about biofeedback are also furnished for the patient to read. A clear understanding of biofeedback is very important for establishing the correct

EMG FEEDBACK EXERCISE

RELAXATION OF FACIAL AREA WITH NECK, SHOULDERS AND UPPER BACK

TIME: 4 - 5 MINUTES

LET ALL YOUR MUSCLES GO LOOSE AND HEAVY. JUST SETTLE BACK QUIETLY AND COMFORTABLE. WRINKLE UP YOUR FOREHEAD NOW; WRINKLE AND SMOOTH IT OUT. PICTURE THE ENTIRE FOREHEAD AND SCALP BECOMING SMOOTHER AS THE RELAXATION INCREASES....NOW FROWN AND CREASE YOUR BROWS AND STUDY THE TENSION....LET GO OF THE TENSION AGAIN. SMOOTH OUT THE FOREHEAD ONCE MORE.... NOW, CLOSE YOUR EYES TIGHTER AND TIGHTER. FEEL THE TENSION.... AND RELAX YOUR EYES. KEEP YOUR EYES CLOSED, GENTLY, COMFORTABLY, AND NOTICE THE RELAXATION....NOW CLENCH YOUR JAWS, BITE YOUR TEETH TOGETHER; STUDY THE TENSION THROUGHOUT THE JAWS.... RELAX YOUR JAWS NOW. LET YOUR LIPS PART SLIGHTLY....APPRECIATE THE RELAXATION....NOW PRESS YOUR TONGUE HARD AGAINST THE ROOF OF YOUR MOUTH. LOOK FOR THE TENSION....ALL RIGHT, LET YOUR TONGUE RETURN TO A COMFORTABLE AND RELAXED POSITION....NOW PURSE YOUR LIPS, PRESS YOUR LIPS TOGETHER TIGHTER AND TIGHTER.... RELAX THE LIPS. NOTE THE CONTRAST BETWEEN TENSION AND RELAXATION. FEEL THE RELAXATION ALL OVER YOUR FACE, ALL OVER YOUR FOREHEAD AND SCALP, EYES, JAWS, LIPS,TONGUE, AND YOUR NECK MUSCLES. PRESS YOUR HEAD BACK AS FAR AS IT CAN GO AND FEEL THE TENSION IN THE NECK; ROLL IT TO THE RIGHT AND FEEL THE TENSION SHIFT; NOW ROLL IT TO THE LEFT. STRAIGHTEN YOUR HEAD AND BRING IT FORWARD AND PRESS YOUR CHIN AGAINST YOUR CHEST. LET YOUR HEAD RETURN TO A COMFORTABLE POSITION, AND STUDY THE RELAXATION. LET THE RELAXATION DEVELOP....SHRUG YOUR SHOULDERS RIGHT UP. HOLD THE TENSION....DROP YOUR SHOULDERS AND FEEL THE RELAXATION. NECK AND SHOULDERS RELAXED....SHRUG YOUR SHOULDERS AGAIN AND MOVE THEM AROUND. BRING YOUR SHOULDERS UP AND FORWARD AND BACK. FEEL THE TENSION IN YOUR SHOULDERS AND IN YOUR UPPER BACK.... DROP YOUR SHOULDERS ONCE MORE AND RELAX. LET THE RELAXATION SPREAD DEEP INTO THE SHOULDERS, RIGHT INTO YOUR BACK MUSCLES; RELAX YOUR NECK AND THROAT, AND YOUR JAWS AND OTHER FACIAL AREAS AS THE PURE RELAXATION TAKES OVER AND GROWS DEEPER.... DEEPER....EVER DEEPER.

Figure 13.6.

cognitive orientation of the patient. The therapist also instructs the patient in the use of the temperature or the EMG trainer. At this visit, a one-to-one relationship is established between therapist and patient.

On follow-up visits, the therapist should report any problems to the physician. This is important so that the physician can keep in close touch with the patient's progress. The therapist also plays a key role by encouraging the patient, emphasizing and praising all progress and helping to stimulate motivation.

This is a key part in any effective therapy program.

Goals are not generalized, with the training continued on an individual basis. External factors affecting training are identified. For example, patients may be told that warm hands before the session may result in a small increase on the temperature monitor. The patients are assisted in recognizing stress points, any patterns in headaches and in reviewing and redesigning biofeedback techniques. All those functions require careful diligent attention from the therapist. Obviously, the attitude of the therapist can affect the patient's success. A relaxed manner is necessary, along with confidence in the use of various instruments. Flexibility in the various techniques will help in each patient's therapy. Firmness with the patients is also required in stressing home practice and in maintaining high motivational levels.

OUTCOME AUDIT OF BIOFEEDBACK

The results of a survey of patients treated at the Diamond Headache Clinic are reported below (Diamond et al., 1978; Diamond et al., 1979; Diamond and Franklin, 1975). A questionnaire, asking their opinion about the effectiveness of the therapy, was mailed to the 556 patients instructed in both electromyographic and temperature feedback over the past 5 years. Of these patients, 413 answered the questionnaire. Their ages ranged between 9 and 71, with an average age of 36 years. The distribution of types of headache was: 115 patients had migraine, 15 had muscle contraction headache and 283 had mixed muscle contraction and migraine headache. They terminated their training period between 3 and 62 months ago. Of 413 patients, 120 (29%) thought that biofeedback did not help their headaches, 133 (32%) noted transitory improvement, and 160 (39%) permanent relief. The patients with transitory improvement did benefit from 1 to 36 months, with an average of 9.5 months. The patients permanently improved have done well from 4 to 52 months, with an average of 25 months. Seventy-one percent of the patients believed that the technique was helpful for headaches.

Over a 30 month period, 32 patients between the ages of 9 and 18 years were started on the biofeedback program. The results were very promising when using a combination of autogenic phrases and progressive relaxation exercises at home and temperature and EMG feedback training at the Clinic. Only 2 patients had poor response and both had an underlying depression. The data has shown that biofeedback training is an excellent tool in the treatment of childhood migraine (Diamond and Franklin, 1975).

OPERANT CONDITIONING

Further support for the effectiveness of autogenic-biofeedback training comes indirectly from the recent work of Fordyce concerning chronic pain. Fordyce (1974) has shown that there are two sets of factors influencing chronic pain: 1) the organic factors and 2) the learning or conditioning factors. The former involves the traditional disease model perspectives, whereas the latter is much more complex and in many ways more difficult to recognize and to treat. These learning factors can promote and maintain a pain habit. Pain of this nature is referred to as "operant pain."

The basic idea here is that, if the environmental consequences which occur either before, during or after the onset of pain are consistent enough to constitute a pattern, the occurrence of those consequences may be sufficient to bring about pain even after the organic factors have been eliminated.

Probably the most significant learning factor is the way people who are important to the patient react to his behavior while he is experiencing pain. If excessive family attention or extra physician concern is shown toward him when he hurts, then these elements of their behavior become contingent on his being in pain. For example, a spouse may be extra-loving, or the physician may give the patient extra time and attention and prescribe rest and medication. These reactions become the environmental consequences of his being in pain. They happen when he hurts and do not happen when he is well. This systematic set of environmental consequences to pain behavior may prove sufficient to maintain pain (or, as in our case, headaches) even after the original organic factor is gone.

Almost all chronic headache patients will display some degree of operant or learned pain. Since learned pain exists because of the automatic effects of learning, it can be reduced only by following a systematic learning or "unlearning" process. We attempt to explain to the patient and his family about learned or operant pain. This is done by carrying out the following objectives: 1) We reduce pain behavior by withdrawing any positive reinforcement form of behavior. 2) We give positive reinforcement for increased activity and when the patient is feeling well. 3) We attempt to retrain the family unit to reinforce well behavior and to avoid reinforcement of pain behavior. 4) If the patient has a pain or headache syndrome which has a basis for treatment, the organic or treatable factors are corrected so that the operant behavior therapy can also be effective.

CONDITIONED REFLEXES AND MIGRAINE

Specific reflexes associated with behavioral responses in man are few in number. The orienting reflex can be defined as the initial response of the organism to any form of stimulus. According to Pavlov (1927), orienting responses alert and prepare the appropriate sensory systems for the information which is to be received (Table 13.1). When high-intensity stimuli, especially pain, are presented, the orienting reflex is replaced by the defensive reflex, described by Sokolov (1963).

Vasomotor changes accompanying the orienting reflex include vascular constriction in the hands, with vasodilatation at the forehead. The vasomotor responses of a defensive reflex are vasoconstrictive at both sites.

Migraine is considered a neurogenic vasomotor disorder which manifests itself by episodic vasospasms within the internal and external carotid artery beds. Migraine therapy is limited to empirical attempts aimed at the prevention or interruption of the chain of migrainous events or to the alleviation of symptoms. Thus, the current status of migraine drug therapy is not entirely satisfactory and new therapeutic modalities are being sought.

A fortuitous observation made at the Menninger Clinic suggested that training migraine sufferers to raise the temperature in their hands not only enabled them to abort imminent attacks but also led to a reduction in the incidence and intensity of attacks. The mechanism of this phenomenon remains conjectural. It is difficult to study the pathophysiology of migraine because of its elusive manifestations and lack of an animal model. Yet, the chance of discovery of the therapeutic efficacy of volitional vasodilation in the extremities requires at least a hypothetical explanation.

Since migraine is a vasomotor disorder, it is reasonable to assume that whatever mechanism is involved in the modification of an attack would ultimately be related to some hemodynamic change. It could not be simply a vasodilation of the hands, or migraine could be treated by submerging the hands in hot water—a technique known to be therapeutically inefficient except when part of a learned relaxational ceremonial.

Table 13.1. Orienting Response

"What is it?"
The first response of the organism to a sensory stimulus
Muscular activity (ears, eyes)
Salivation
Sweating
Autonomic components
Peripheral vascular constriction
Central vascular dilation
Pupillary dilation
Electrodermal
Decreased skin resistance
Cardiac acceleration
Central nervous system
Desynchronization of alpha activity
Elaboration of evoked responses

Previously we found that, in normal subjects, heating of hands produced total vasodilation both in the extremities and in the frontotemporal region (Sovak et al., 1978). In the same subjects, trained to increase volitionally their digital pulse volume, we found in their upper extremities a total (cutaneous and muscular) vasodilation which coincided with vasoconstriction both in superficial temporal and supraorbital artery beds and a reduction in cardiac rate.

Our later results showed that patients who learned this technique improved with respect to migraine control. We believe that this improvement is related to an alteration in autonomic nervous system activity, a resetting of the balance in that system, with a tendency to decrease sympathetic activity.

In addition to the obvious therapeutic implications of these data, they also contain subtle clues regarding vasomotor abnormalities in migraine and the capacity of migraineurs to influence willfully the activity of their autonomic nervous system. It became obvious that patients with migraine cannot alter their vasomotor responses in the manner of "normal" controls. Even those who do improve with respect to headache incidence cannot duplicate the vasomotor performance of persons without headache. Furthermore, since we know that migraine is at least a familial illness (if not hereditary), the data suggest that this incapacity to alter autonomic functions is a fundamental character of these patients.

The new vasomotor reflex employed by these patients who learn to control their headaches is of considerable interest and has not been described before. To recapitulate, learned dilatation of the peripheral blood vessels of the hand and arm evokes reduced blood flow in the area of the supraorbital and superficial temporal arteries (Table 13.1). The character of this reflex is the antithesis of the orienting reflex, which is a reflex of vigilance produced by a novel situation depending upon the stress involved (Table 13.2). This new reflex can be considered therefore as an adaptation-relaxation reflex. As such, and as postulated in this section, it represents a retraining of the autonomic nervous system to produce a reduction in sympathetic tone. We suggest that this learned adaptation-relaxation reflex may be far more useful than in the relatively narrow context of headache. Similar biofeedback training could be employed in any one of a host of "psychosomatic" and other psychiatric conditions characterized by enhanced sympathetic responsiveness.

These studies suggest also that the volitional higher nervous functions can be used to alter reflex or autonomic nervous responses, that new reflex patterns can be learned or augmented, but that often the new knowledge is incomplete, or only partially learned or the old reflex patterns can be altered to only a finite extent. Further, in our experience, the subject must constantly reproduce the new reflex; it must be reinforced or it will soon be forgotten or, more likely, the inherent primitive older reflex patterns will gain ascendency once again.

Table 13.2. Vasomotor Alterations Reflexology

Pavlov (orienting)	Vasoconstriction	Vasodilation
Sokolov (defensive)	Vasoconstriction	Vasoconstriction
Adaptation-relaxation *	Vasodilation	Vasoconstriction

* Adaptation-relaxation reflex is antithesis of orienting reflex.

References

Budzynski T, Stoyva J, Adler C (1970) Feedback-induced muscle relaxation: Application to tension headache. *Behav Ther Exp Psychol 1*:205.

Diamond S, Franklin M (1975) Autogenic training with biofeedback in the treatment of children with migraine. *Proceedings of Third Congress of the International College of Psychosomatic Medicine*, Second International Symposium of Autogenic Therapy, Rome, Italy, September 16–20, 1975.

Diamond S, Diamond-Falk J, and DeVeno T (1978) Biofeedback in the treatment of vascular headache (Task Force Report). *Biofeedback Self Regul 3*:385–408.

Diamond S, Medina JL, Diamond-Falk J, DeVeno T (1979) The value of biofeedback in the treatment of chronic headache: A five-year retrospective study. *Headache 19*:90.

Fordyce WE (1976) *Behavioral Methods for Chronic Pain and Illness*. St. Louis, CV Mosby.

Pavlov IP (1927) *Conditioned Reflexes*, translated by Anrep GV. New York, Oxford University Press.

Sargent JD, Green EE, Walters ED (1972) The use of autogenic feedback training in a pilot study of migraine and tension headaches. *Headache 12*:120.

Sokolov EN (1963) Higher nervous functions: The orienting reflex. *Annu Rev Physiol 25*:545–580.

Sovak M, Kunzel M, Sternbach RA, et al. (1978) Is volitional manipulation of hemodynamics a valid rationale for biofeedback therapy of migraine? *Headache 18*:197–202.

14

An Atlas of Headache Types

Frank Netter, M.D.

Migraine

A. The aura

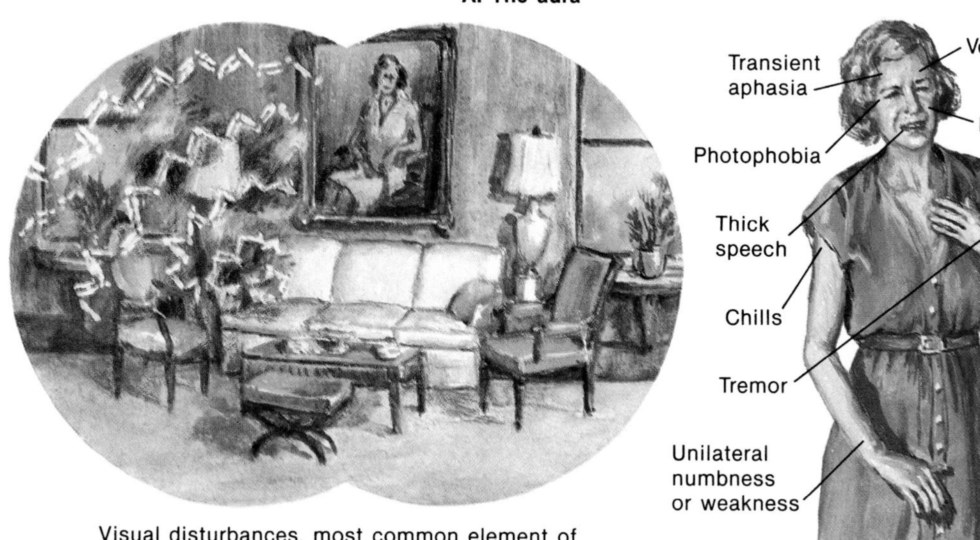

Visual disturbances, most common element of migraine aura: blurred cloudy vision, scotomata, scintillating zigzag lines (fortification spectrum), flashes of light, etc.

Transient aphasia

Vertigo

Pallor

Photophobia

Thick speech

Chills

Tremor

Unilateral numbness or weakness

Some other manifestations of the aura, which may occur individually or in combination

---

B. The attack

Severe, throbbing headache; unilateral at first but may spread to opposite side

Confusion, poor memory, loss of concentration

Tense, irritable, hostile

"Sonophobia"

Local erythema may be present

Photophobia

F. Netter M.D.

Speaks in low voice to avoid aggravating pain

Pallor, perspiration

Vomiting may occur

Plate 14.1

Biochemistry of Migraine

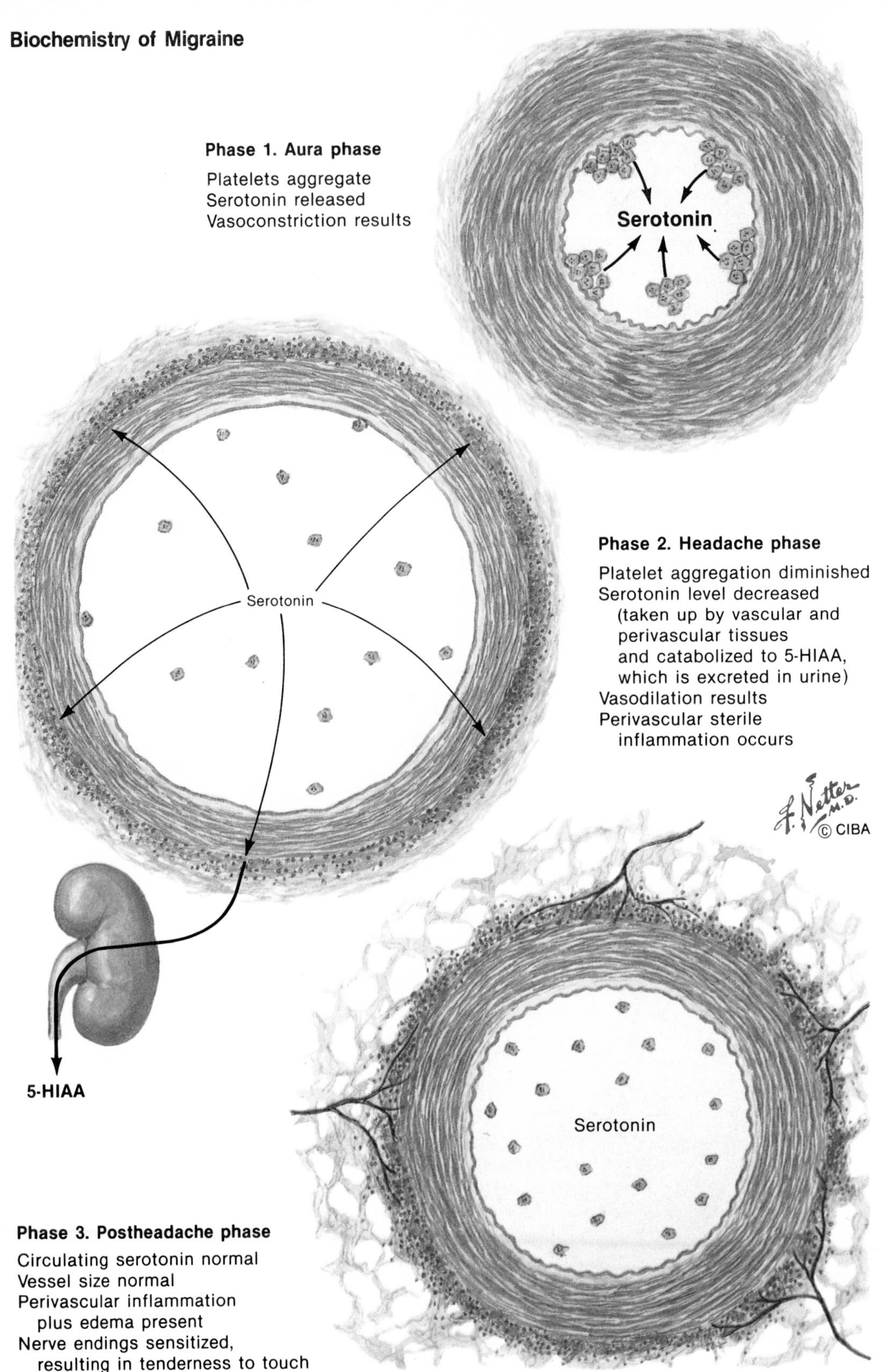

Plate 14.2

Giant Cell Arteritis, Polymyalgia Rheumatica

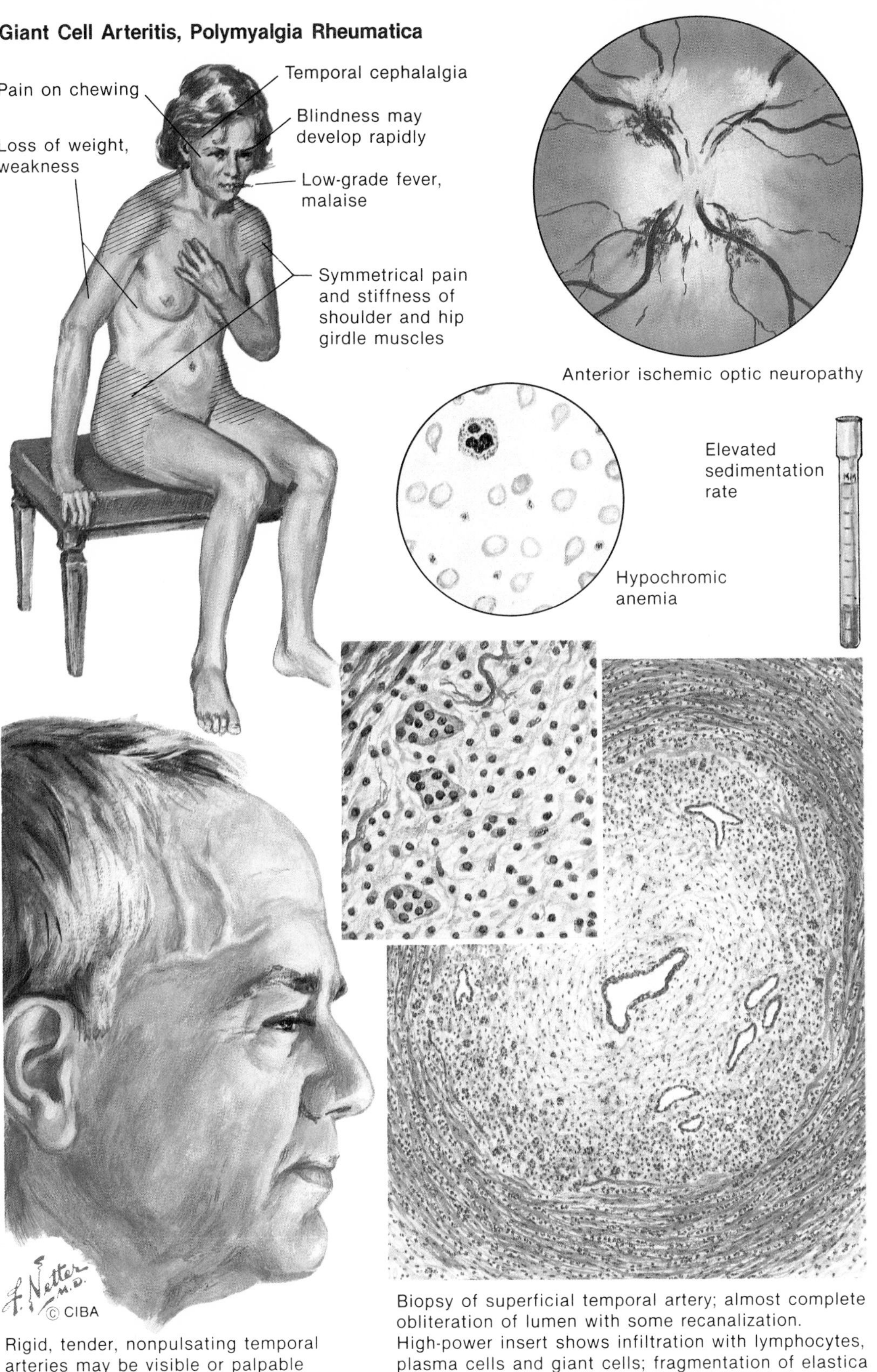

Rigid, tender, nonpulsating temporal arteries may be visible or palpable

Biopsy of superficial temporal artery; almost complete obliteration of lumen with some recanalization. High-power insert shows infiltration with lymphocytes, plasma cells and giant cells; fragmentation of elastica

Plate 14.7

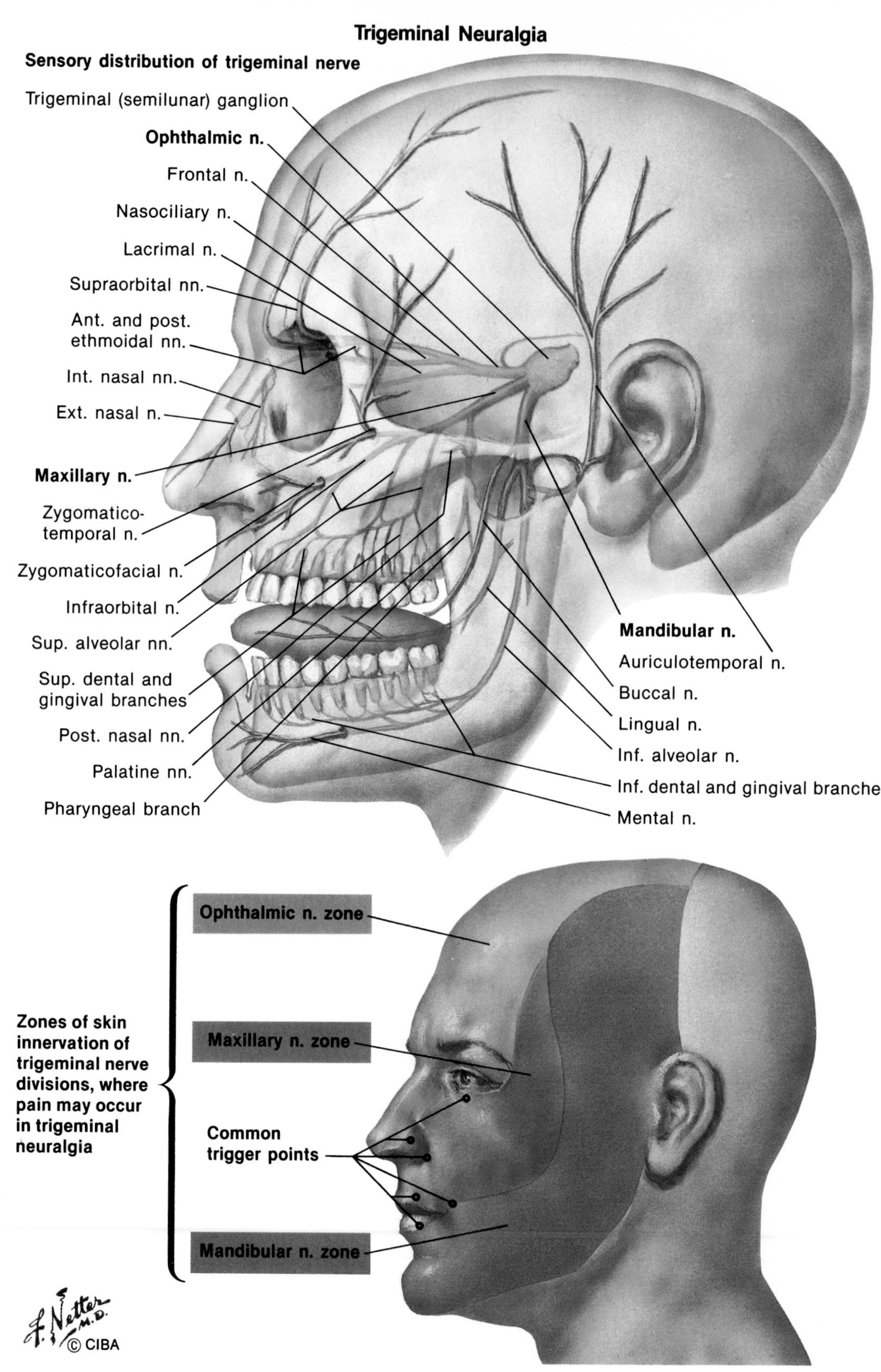
Trigeminal Neuralgia
Sensory distribution of trigeminal nerve
Trigeminal (semilunar) ganglion
Ophthalmic n.
Frontal n.
Nasociliary n.
Lacrimal n.
Supraorbital nn.
Ant. and post. ethmoidal nn.
Int. nasal nn.
Ext. nasal n.
Maxillary n.
Zygomatico-temporal n.
Zygomaticofacial n.
Infraorbital n.
Sup. alveolar nn.
Sup. dental and gingival branches
Post. nasal nn.
Palatine nn.
Pharyngeal branch
Mandibular n.
Auriculotemporal n.
Buccal n.
Lingual n.
Inf. alveolar n.
Inf. dental and gingival branches
Mental n.
Ophthalmic n. zone
Maxillary n. zone
Common trigger points
Mandibular n. zone
Zones of skin innervation of trigeminal nerve divisions, where pain may occur in trigeminal neuralgia
F. Netter M.D.
© CIBA

Plate 14.8

Additional Bibliography

Adams F: Extant Works of Aretaeus the Cappadocian. London, The Sydenham Society, 1856

Alestig K, Barr J: Giant-cell arteritis. Lancet 1:1228, 1963

Anthony M, Hinterberger H, Lance JW: Plasma serotonin in migraine and stress. Arch Neurol 16:544, 1967

Appenzeller O: Reflex vasomotor function: Clinical and experimental studies in migraine. Res Clin Stud Headache 6:160–166, 1978

Aurelianus C: Liber 1. De Capitis Passione, quam Graeci Cephalaean Nominant: Medici Antiqui Omnes Qui Latinis, etc. Venetiis 4:249, 1547

Background to Migraine: Proceedings. 1st Symposium on Migraine. London, 1966. R. Smith, ed. New York, Springer-Verlag, 1967

Background to Migraine: Proceedings. 2nd Symposium on Migraine. London, 1967. R. Smith, ed. New York, Springer-Verlag, 1969

Background to Migraine: Proceedings. 3rd Symposium on Migraine. London, 1969. AL Cochrane, ed. New York, Springer-Verlag, 1970

Barcroft JC, Binger CA, Bock AV, et al: Observations upon the effect of high altitude on the physiological process of the human body. Phil Trans R Soc (Lond) Ser B 211:351, 1922

Behnke, AR: Problems in the treatment of decompression sickness (and traumatic air embolism). Ann NY Acad Sci 117:843–859, 1965

Blom S: Tic douloureux treated with a new anticonvulsant. Arch Neurol 9:285, 1963

Brodie BB, Shore PA: A concept for the role of serotonin and norepinephrine as chemical mediators in the brain. Ann NY Acad Sci 66: 631, 1957

Carliner NH, Denune DL, Finch CS, Goldberg LI: Sodium nitroprusside treatment of ergotamine-induced peripheral ischemia. JAMA 227:308, 1974

Catino D: Ten migraine equivalents. Headache 5:1, 1965

Couch JR, Hassanein RS: Platelet aggregability in migraine and relation of aggregability to clinical aspects of migraine. Neurology 26:348, 1976.

Curzon G, Theaker P, Phillips BJ: Excretion of 5-hydroxyindole acetic acid in migraine. J Neurol Neurosurg Psychiatry 29:85, 1966

Dalessio DJ: On migraine headache: Serotonin and serotonin antagonism. JAMA 181:318, 1962

Dalessio DJ: Wolff's Headache and Other Head Pain, ed 3. New York, Oxford University Press, 1972

Dalessio DJ: Wolff's Headache and Other Head Pain, ed 4. New York, Oxford University Press, 1980

Dalessio DJ: Effort migraine. Headache 14:53, 1974

Dalessio DJ: Mechanisms of headache. Med Clin North Am 62:429–442, 1978

Dalessio DJ, Kunzel M, Sternbach RA, Sovak M.: Conditioned adaptation-relaxation reflex in migraine therapy. JAMA 242:2102–2104, 1979

Dalsgaard-Nielsen T, Genefke IK: Serotonin release and uptake in platelets from healthy persons and migraine patients in attack-free intervals. Headache 14:26, 1974

Diamond S, Baltes BJ: Management of headache by the family physician. Am Fam Physician 5:68–76, 1972

Diamond S, Medina JL: The headache history—the key to diagnosis. In Pathogenesis and Treatment of Headache. O Appenzeller, ed. Spectrum Publications, New York, 1976

Diamond S, Medina JL, Diamond-Falk J, DeVeno T: The value of biofeedback in the treatment of chronic headache: A five-year retrospective study. Headache 19:90–96, 1979

Dukes HT, Vieth RG: Cerebral arteriography during migraine prodrome and headache. Neurology 14:636, 1964

Edmeads J, Hachinski VC, Norris JW: Ergotamine and the cerebral circulation. Hemicrania 7:6, 1976

Ekbom K: Studies on cluster headache. Sundbyberg, Sweden, Solna Tryckeri AB, 1970

Ekbom K: Some observations on pain in cluster headache. Headache 14:219–225, 1975

Engel GL, Webb JP, Ferris EB, et al: A migraine-like syndrome complicating decompression sickness. War Med 5:304–314, 1944

Erde AE, Edmonds C: Decompression sickness: A clinical series. J Occupat Med 17:324, 1975

Fog M: Cerebral circulation. 1. Reaction of pial arteries to epinephrine by direct application and by intravenous injection. Arch Neurol Psychiatry 41:109, 1939

Fordyce WE: Recent Advances on Pain: Pathophysiology and Clinical Aspects. JJ Bonica, P Procacci, CA Pagni, eds. Springfield, Ill., Charles C Thomas, 1974, pp. 299–312

Forward SA, Landowne M, Follansbee JN, Hansen JE: Effect of acetazolamide on acute mountain sickness. N Engl J Med 279:839, 1968

Friedman AP: Migraine. Med Clin North Am 62:481–494, 1978

Friedman AP, Merritt HH: Treatment of headache. JAMA 143:111, 1957

Galen: De Compositione Medicamentorum Secundum Locos. In: Opera Omnia. Ed. Kuhn. Lipsiae: C. Cnoblochii. Vol 12, book 2, Cap. III (De hemicrania), 1826, p 591

Glover V, Sandler M, Grant E, Rose FC, Orton D, Wilkinson M, Stevens D: Transitory decrease in platelet monoamine oxidase activity during migraine attacks. Lancet 1:391, 1977

Graham JR, Wolff HG: Mechanism of migraine headache and action of ergotamine tartrate. Arch Neurol Psychiatry 39:737, 1938

Greenblatt SH: Post-traumatic transient cerebral blindness. JAMA 225:1073, 1973

Hachinski VC, Norris JW, Cooper PW, Edmeads JG: Ergotamine tartrate and cerebral blood flow. Can J Neurol Sci 2:333, 1975

Headache Update, Organon Labs, No's 1, 2, 3, 4, 1976–1977

Hilton BP, Cumings JN: 5-Hydroxytryptamine levels and platelet aggregation responses in subjects with acute migraine. J Neurol Neurosurg Psychiatry 35:505, 1972

Hilton BP, Cumings JN: An assessment of platelet aggregation induced by 5-hydroxytryptamine. J Clin Pathol 24:250, 1971

Hirofumi M, Chun HL, Lee CC, Pasquale AC, Christie JH: Reliability of computed tomography: Correlation with neuropathologic findings. Am J Roentgenol 128:795–798, 1977

Hounsfield GN: Computerized transverse axial scanning

(tomography); Part I. Description of system. Br J Radiol 46:1016–1022, 1973

Houston CS: High altitude illness. JAMA 236:2193–2195, 1976

Huckman MS, Grainer LS, Clasen RC: The normal computed tomogram. Semin Roentgenol 12:27–38, 1977

Ingvar DH: Pain in the brain—and migraine. Hemicrania 7:2, 1976

Jannetta PJ: Observations on the etiology of trigeminal neuralgia, hemifacial spasm, acoustic nerve dysfunction and glossopharyngeal neuralgia: Definitive microsurgical treatment and results in 117 patients. Neurochirurgia 20:145–154, 1977

Jay GW, Tomasi LG: Pediatric headaches: A one-year retrospective analysis. Headache 21:5–9, 1981

Kerr FWL: The etiology of trigeminal neuralgia. Arch Neurol 8:15, 1963

Koppman JW, McDonald RD, Kunzel MG: Voluntary regulation of temporal artery diameter by migraine patients. Headache 14(3):133, 1974

Kudrow L: Comparative results of prednisone, methysergide, and lithium therapy in cluster headache. Abstracts, International Symposium, London, Migraine Trust, Sept. 16–17, 1976

Kudrow L: Cluster headache: Diagnosis and management. Headache 19:142–150, 1979

Kugelberg E, Lindblom U: The mechanism of pain in trigeminal neuralgia. J Neurol Neurosurg Psychiatry 22:36, 1959

Lance JW: The Mechanism and Management of Headache. London, Butterworth & Co (Publishers) Ltd, 1969

Lance JW: Migraine. In The Mechanism and Management of Headache, ed 2. London, Butterworth & Co, 1973

Lance JW: Pattern recognition from the history. In Mechanisms and Management of Headache. London, Butterworth & Co., 1978

Lance JW, Anthony M, Gonski A: Serotonin, the carotid body, and cranial vessels in migraine. Arch Neurol 16:553, 1967

Lance JW, Curran DA: Treatment of chronic tension headache. Lancet 1:1236, 1964

Lassen NA, Ingvar DH: The blood flow of the cerebral cortex determined by Krypton 85. Experientia 17:42, 1961

Lenfant C, Sullivan K: Adaptation to high altitude. N Engl J Med 284:1298, 1971

Lepois C: Selectiorum Observationum. Ludg. Batav.: C Boutestein and JA Langerak. De Hemicrania, pp. 67–77, 1714

Li CL, Ahlberg H, Lansdell MA, et al: Acupuncture and hypnosis: Effects on induced pain. Exp Neurol 49:272–280, 1975

Liang GC, Simkin P, Mannik M: Immunoglobulins in temporal arteritis. Ann Intern Med 81:19, 1974

Liveing E: On Megrim. Sick-headache and Some Allied Disorders. London, Churchill, 1873

Lovshin LL: Treatment of histaminic cephalalgia with methysergide. Dis Nerv Syst 24:3, 1963

Martin MJ: Psychogenic factors—Headache. Med Clin North Am 62:559–570, 1978

Mathew N: Prophylaxis of migraine and mixed headache. A randomized controlled study. Headache 21:105, 1981

Mathew N: Indomethacin responsive headache syndromes. Headache 21:147, 1981

Mathew NT, Hrastnick F, Meyer JS: Regional cerebral blood flow in the diagnosis of vascular headache. Headache 15:252, 1976

Matthews WB: Footballer's migraine. Br Med J 2:326–327, 1972

Medina JL, Diamond S: Proceedings of the Third International Symposium of the Migraine Trust. Belmont, Calif., Pitman Medical, in press, 1982

Meyer JS, Yoshida K, Sakamoto K: Autonomic control of cerebral blood flow measured by electromagnetic flowmeters. Neurology 17:638, 1967

Miller NE: Learning of visceral and glandular responses. Science 163:434, 1969

Morley TP: The place of peripheral and subtemporal ablative operations in the treatment of trigeminal neuralgia. Clin Neurosurg 24:550, 1977

Nelson E, Rennels M: Neuromuscular contact in intracranial arteries of the cat. Science 167:301, 1970

Nielsen KC, Owman C: Adrenergic innervation of pial arteries related to the circle of Willis in the cat. Brain Res 6:773, 1967

Nielsen KC, Owman C: Contractile response and amine receptor mechanisms in isolated middle cerebral artery of the cat. Brain Res 27:33, 1971

Norris JW, Hachinski VC, Cooper PW: Changes in cerebral blood flow during a migraine attack. Br Med J 3:676, 1975

Norris JW, Hachinski VC, Cooper PW: Cerebral blood flow changes in cluster headache. Acta Neurol Scand 54:371, 1976

Onel Y, Friedman AP, Grossman J: Muscle blood flow studies in muscle contraction headaches. Neurology 11:935, 1961

Ostfeld AM, Wolff HG: Studies on headache: Arterenol (norepinephrine) and vascular headache of the migraine type. Arch Neurol Psychiatry 74:131, 1955

Pearce J: Migraine: Clinical Features, Mechanisms, and Management. Springfield, Ill. Charles C Thomas, 1969

Pearce JMS: Chronic migrainous neuralgia. A variant of cluster headache. Brain 103:149–150, 1980

Phelps ME, Kuhl DE, Mazziotta JC: Metabolic mapping of the brain's response to visual stimulation: Studies in humans. Science 211:1445–1448, 1981

Pickering GW: Experimental observations on headache. Br Med J 1:4087, 1939

Pilowsky I: Dimensions of hypochondriasis. Br J Psychiatry 113:89–93, 1967

Prensky AL, Sommer D: Diagnosis and treatment of migraine in children. Neurology 29:506–510, 1979

Proceedings of the International Headache Symposium, Elsinore, Denmark, May 16–18, 1971; DJ Dalessio, T Dalsgaard-Nielsen, S Diamond, eds. Basel, Switzerland, Sandoz Ltd

Raskin NH, Schwartz RK: Prophylaxis of migraine—A long-term controlled study. Neurology 30:418, 1980

Robb LG: Severe vasospasm following ergot administration. West J Med 123:231, 1975

Rothner AD: Headache in children: A review. Headache 18:169–175, 1978

Sacks OW: Migraine, the Evolution of a Common Disorder. Berkeley, University of California Press, 1970

Sandler M, Youdim MBH, Hanington E: A phenylethylamine oxidising defect in migraine. Nature 250:335, 1974

Sandler M, Youdim MBH, Southgate J, Hanington E: The role of tyramine in migraine: Some possible biochemical mechanisms, In Background to Migraine, Third Migraine Symposium. AL Cochrane, ed. London, Heinemann, 1970, p. 103

Saper J: Migraine: I. Classification and pathogenesis. II. Treatment. JAMA 239:2380–2383, 2480–2484, 1978

Schildkraut JJ, Kety SS: Biogenic amines and emotion. Science 156:21, 1967

Schildkraut JJ, Schanberg SM, Breese GR, et al.: Norepinephrine metabolism and drugs used in the affective disorders: A possible mechanism of action. Am J Psychiatry 124:56, 1967

Schiller F: The migraine tradition. Bull Hist Med 49:1, 1975

Segal J: Biofeedback as a medical treatment. JAMA 232:179, 1975.

Sicuteri F: Mast cells and their active substances: Their role in the pathogenesis of migraine. Headache 3:86, 1963

Sicuteri F: Vasoneuractive substances in migraine. Headache 6:109, 1966

Sicuteri F, Anselmi B, et al: Morphine-like factors in CSF of headache patients. In The Endorphins. E Costa and M Trabucchi, eds. New York, Raven Press, 1978

Sicuteri F, Buffoni F, Anselmi B, Bel Bianco PL: An enzyme (MAO) defect on the platelets in migraine. Res Clin Stud Headache 3:245, 1972

Sicuteri F, Testi A, Anselmi B: Biochemical investigations in headache. Int Arch Allergy Appl Immunol 19:55, 1961

Simard D, Paulson OB: Cerebral vasomotor paralysis during migraine attack. Arch Neurol 29:207, 1973

Sjaastad O: Introduction: Chronic Paroxysmal Hemicrania. Proceedings The Bergen Migraine Symposium, Joint Meeting American Association for the Study of Headache and Scandinavian Migraine Society, Bergen, Norway, June 4–6, 1975

Sjaastad O, Dale I: Evidence for a new treatable headache entity. Headache 14:105–108, 1974

Skinhoj E: Hemodynamic studies within the brain during migraine. Arch Neurol 29:95, 1973

Skinhoj E, Paulson OB: Regional blood flow in internal carotid distribution during migraine attack. Br Med J 3:569, 1969

Smith I, Kellow AH, Hanington E: Tyramine metabolism in dietary migraine. In Background to Migraine, Third British Migraine Symposium, London, Heinemann, 1970

Sokolav EN: Perception and the conditioned reflex. 330, Moscow University Press, 1958.

Sovak M, Fronek A, Helland DR, Doyle R: Effects of vasomotor changes in the upper extremities on the hemodynamics of the carotid arterial beds. A possible mechanism of biofeedback therapy of migraine. Proceedings of the San Diego Biomedical Meeting, vol. 15. Academic Press, New York, 1976, p. 363

Sternbach R, Deems LM, Timmermans G, Huey L: On the sensitivity of the tourniquet pain test. Pain 3:105, 1977

Symonds CP: Cough headache. Brain 79:557, 1956

Timmermans G, Sternbach RA: Factors of human chronic pain: An analysis of personality and pain reaction variables. Science 184:806, 1974

Tissot SAD: Traité des nerfs et de leurs maladies. Lausanne, Paris, 1873

Walker AE: Chronic post-traumatic headache. Headache 5:67, 1965

Welch KMA, Chabi E, Bartosh L, Achar US, Meyer JS: Cerebrospinal fluid gamma aminobutyric acid levels in migraine. Br Med J 3:516, 1975

Welch KMA, Nell J, Chabi E, Matthew NT, Neblett CR, Meyer JS: Cyclic nucleotide studies in migraine. Neurology 26:380, 1976

Woolf AL, Quest IA: Fatal infarction of the brain in migraine. Br Med J 1:225, 1964

Ziegler D: Tension headache. Med Clin North Am 62:495–505, 1978

Zweifach BW: Microcirculatory aspects of tissue injury. Ann NY Acad Sci 116:831, 1964

Index

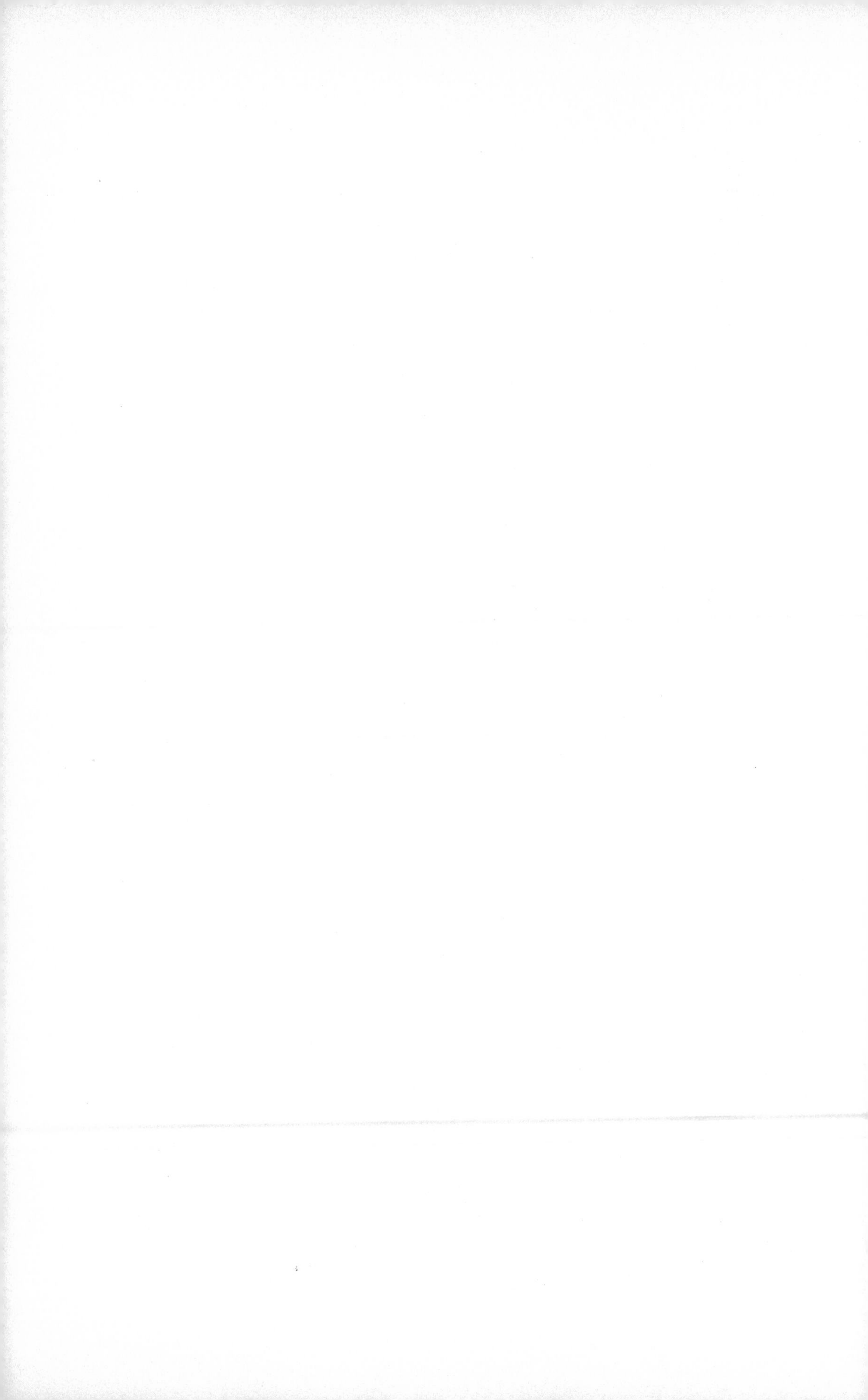